OUT OF ISOLATION
A Charity Anthology

Edited by Susie Coreth

UNICORN

Published by Unicorn Publishing Group
Charleston Studio
Meadow Business Centre
Lewes BN8 5RW
www.unicornpublishing.org

A CIP record for this book is available from the British Library

ISBN 978-1-914414-31-2

10 9 8 7 6 5 4 3 2 1

Cover design Felicity Price-Smith
Typeset by Vivian Head

Printed in Malta by Gutenberg Press Ltd

Contents

– Introduction –

The idea for *Out of Isolation* came to me in the winter of 2020, when the UK went from a second lockdown to a third, with some semblance of Christmas and the turning of a new year in the middle. Having spent the autumn months tentatively seeing friends and family again, it struck me how often our conversations would turn from describing our different attempts at lockdown entertainment to an honest reflection on moments when they or someone they were close to had found it really, really hard. Almost every conversation I was having included discussion about an increased struggle with depression and anxiety. It was clear how much the pandemic was affecting people's mental health and therefore I could not help but think about the increased pressure that mental health charities must be under.

Shout 85258 is an important charity that uses a free, 24/7 text messaging support service for anyone in the UK who is struggling to cope. What I think is so brilliant about Shout is that someone can get confidential support in any place, at any time, even if they are unable to find a private space to do so. At times of vulnerability, when one might not feel able or comfortable discussing a situation out loud, the ability to access help quietly and privately is essential. I hope that through this anthology, we can raise some money for Shout 85258 to help those who need it and spread a wider awareness of this crucial service. You can find more information about the charity on p. xx

Alongside raising much needed finances, with *Out of Isolation* I wanted to create something that is a genuinely interesting read; a book you can dip into and discover something unexpected. As an avid reader, I find comfort, catharsis and escape in others' writing. I spent a lot of my time over the pandemic reading books that had long been on my bookshelf. They provided a much-needed break from my own thoughts and, judging by the amount of reading clubs I saw on social media, they did for many others too.

As a writer, I was intrigued by what other writers had been working on during the continued months of pandemic inertia. Did they, like me for much of 2020, find themselves stifled with writer's block? Did they pen something outside of their usual form or style? Were they writing something specific, perhaps something previously planned, or were their words and creativity fuelled by the situation? Were their scribblings about the pandemic or had their minds taken them elsewhere entirely?

What you will see when reading this anthology is that people were writing about all sorts of things: love, horticulture, history, travel, reflections, flight, daily life, pregnancy, humanity, nature and more. Some of the authors have included extracts from books they were working on during 2020, or short stories they wrote in lockdown, or personal diary entries. Some have reflected on their own experience of the pandemic (for which we have included the month they wrote it for context). Dame Carol Ann Duffy kindly allowed me to choose a poem from her *Collected Poems*. *Silver Lining*, which she wrote in 2010 when the ash cloud from the volcanic eruptions in Iceland grounded planes, was on the very first page I opened. The poem immediately struck me as one which could have been written about the pandemic and it felt so poignant to read it in that moment, just as the third lockdown was beginning to ease, that I knew it needed to be included. Its similarity – reflecting on nature and the silver linings we can find when we look out for them – to that of other pieces in this anthology, is a beautiful insight into what we notice when we are forced to stop.

I was amazed by every piece that was sent to me and I will forever be grateful to the authors for giving their time and their words. Each author surprised and delighted me more than I could believe and, in my humble opinion, the collection as a whole, with both its variety and its similarities, provides a fascinating look at creative minds during an intensely challenging time.

I hope you enjoy reading the pieces as much as I did.

Susie Coreth

OLIVIA ACLAND

– Three Stages –

The fear

At the beginning, Covid-19 was seen as a disease that only white people caught. In fact, white people became the disease. I work as a journalist in Goma, a city in eastern Democratic Republic of the Congo, which is sandwiched between a lake and a volcano and nudges the Rwandan border. When the pandemic first struck, it hit Europe harder than Africa.

I get around Goma on a rattling motorbike and as a rare female motorcyclist, I usually receive friendly attention from other drivers. Bashed up minibuses overtake take me and passengers stick their heads out of the window to shout, 'courage ma soeur' and give me thumbs-up signs.

However, in March last year, when I paused at a traffic-clogged roundabout, I only heard the words, 'corona, corona' echoing around me. Men on motorbikes wagged fingers at me and yelled things in Swahili, another language spoken in eastern Congo. Generally, I understood little of their shouts, save two words: 'mzungu' (white person) and 'corona'.

Hundreds of foreign aid workers live in Goma and when some of them received this kind of attention, they started to panic, fearing they might be targeted and attacked. The city is surrounded by 130 armed groups, fighting over land rich in gold and coltan (a metal used in mobile phone batteries). The region has been ravaged by conflict for twenty-five years and rebels often turn their guns on civilians, looting and kidnapping to fund their lives in the bush. In such a volatile environment, matters can turn nasty quickly. 'I worry that people will turn on us, break into our compounds and loot our houses,' my downstairs neighbour, an anxious Frenchman, told me one evening.

Meanwhile, lots of Congolese people were far more worried about the closure of the Rwandan border, prompted by Covid-19. It is one of the busiest crossings in the world. Normally, more than 30,000 petty traders pass through it each day, variously lugging sacks of potatoes and swinging chicken by the feet. A lot of the food consumed in Goma comes from Rwanda, so when the border closed, prices shot up. Staples like rice and beans cost a third more, while salt and bananas were twice as expensive. Although lorries loaded with goods were still allowed to cross, traders had to pay $100 a day to hire them as well as cough up the taxes they were dodging on foot.

'If this confinement continues, then we'll die,' said Claude Bahati, a forty-six-year-old cleaner, slumped on a plastic chair outside a shop. He had been laid off work and was forfeiting his salary of $70 a month. The price hikes also meant that his wife could only afford to buy half of what she used to at the market. 'We used to eat twice a day. Now we only eat once,' he said, 'In the morning when I wake up, my stomach is empty so I drink a lot of water.'

The denial

After some months, cases continued to climb gradually, but the panic that was palpable at the start of the pandemic seemed to dissolve. The border with Rwanda re-opened, people were friendly to me again on my motorbike and, as far as I know, no 'mzungu' (least of all my downstairs neighbour) had their house looted. In fact, people's attitudes seemed to swing the other way. Many Congolese denied that Covid-19 was a problem and refused to take the vaccine.

While leaders at the G7 summit in Cornwall solemnly pledged to donate more vaccines to Africa, vaccination tents in Goma stood empty. When a friend and I turned up to get our shots of the AstraZeneca vaccine, we were the only people there, except for the nurses dishing out the jabs. Rumours circulated that the vaccine made you sterile. Wackier conspiracists whispered that doses had been sent by Westerners who wanted to kill Congolese people and reduce the global population.

There was no campaign to counter these claims. Fake news spread across Facebook and WhatsApp. Few people argued with it. Lots of Congolese simply did not understand the risks of Covid-19, nor the real benefits of the vaccine. If government officials had made an effort to disseminate real information, people would have listened and turned up for their jabs, but they didn't. Flying a million vaccines into a country is just the starting point.

Meanwhile, next door in tiny Rwanda, people were queueing up for their vaccines. The autocratic president, Paul Kagame, had also introduced fierce penalties for those caught flouting Covid rules. Anyone caught walking down the street with their nose sticking out of the top of their face mask would be rounded up by the police and dumped in the stadium all night long. They would sit in plastic seats as recorded messages about safe Covid practices were droned out over loudspeakers. Those caught meeting in groups of more than six would be hauled out of their houses and photographed, with their pictures stuck up on a government website.

As frightening as his methods were, Kagame did manage to contain the pandemic. At least, he did until a load of Congolese people hurried into Rwanda when a volcano erupted in Goma. Many took the virus with them.

The volcano

The first text message came in at around 6.45 pm one Saturday night. 'The volcano is erupting,' wrote an English friend of mine, Alex. I was in the car, heading for dinner at a pizza restaurant, and as I turned a corner I saw the sky, smoky and orange. The lights flickered off across the city as lava, which was leaking out of a fissure and rolling towards Goma, melted electricity pylons.

Mount Nyiragongo, which looms over Goma, last erupted in 2002 and killed over one hundred people in Goma. Remembering the horror, thousands of people panicked and made for the Rwandan border, carrying mattresses on their heads.

I rushed up to a hotel rooftop to get a better view. Alarmed friends were calling me every few minutes and we decided to get together and discuss escape plans. Soon, six of us were huddled together. Those working for NGOs were receiving garbled instructions. 'We need to get across the border at once,' urged one friend after a series of calls with her security manager. Another insisted we should stay put, as opportunistic thieves, possibly armed, were taking advantage of the chaos and attacking cars on the roads. Eventually we split ways, with some heading for the border. I went to a friend's house nearby, which was close to the lake. We hauled a paddleboard out of a cupboard just in case the lava spilled down the hill and we needed to get away across the water.

The next morning, alarmed and exhausted, I headed to Buhene, a district in the north of the city. It had been flattened by molten lava and sulphurous smoke billowed off cooling black rocks. Hundreds of people wandered around on the rubble, lots of them, bizarrely, taking selfies. However, far more desperate were the former residents of the 'quartiere'. One man wearily picked through scraps of metal and examined some scorched pots. He was standing in what used to be his kitchen, he said. He had been out during the blast and his two young children had been at home with his neighbours. He had not been able to find them since. He said he planned to head to a local radio station to tell them where he was. Wearily, he also explained that all his savings had melted inside his house. 'I hope the government will help us with some food or clothes for the time being,' he said, quietly. Thirty-two people died in the blast and around 3,000 houses were destroyed.

After visiting the tragic destruction, I headed to a hotel which had a generator so that I could send my words and photos to the *Economist*. Sitting on the second floor, red-eyed and reeking of sulphur fumes, I ordered a fish and started writing. Moments after opening my laptop, an earthquake shook the building. The waitresses shrieked and ran outside. This was to be the first of 300 earthquakes that we experienced over the next three days.

Volcanologists reckoned that the regular earthquakes meant there might be another eruption, and at 3.00 am on a Thursday morning, the governor of Goma ordered most of the city to evacuate. He said, 'Our current data indicates the presence of magma underneath the urban zone of Goma with an extension under Lake Kivu.' As had happened on Saturday night, people streamed towards the Rwandan border.

I packed a small bag and jumped on my motorbike, heading for the border with a friend. We wove in and out of traffic jams, while people on the pavement carried bundles of clothes on their heads. We waited for two hours at the border in gridlocked traffic, as we left the lakeside, driving to safety in Rwanda's green hills, I noticed that the lake had turned a strange colour. There was a band of greeny-grey water, close to the shore. It could have been a sign of an imminent limnic eruption. This is when the lake explodes because gases have built up in the deep water. It can be caused by earthquakes or lava flows into the lake. If there were a limnic eruption (thankfully they are very rare, the last one happened in Cameroon in 1986), the whole city would be engulfed in a tsunami-like tidal wave, accompanied by a fog of carbon dioxide. Everyone within 25km would probably suffocate and die.

The border was moved 12km into Rwanda, so that people could get away as quickly as possible. Thankfully, the volcano did not erupt again, nor did the lake explode, but there was a major uptick in Covid cases in Rwanda a week later – Goma's fugitives were likely the cause. As the Delta variant tears through Congo and Rwanda, the border has been closed again and curfews reinstated. A Congolese friend called me the other day saying, 'It's got bad, now we want that vaccine, people are dying everywhere.' The vaccines they had have expired and so now the Congolese are sitting tight, waiting for more doses.

– simplicity is beautiful –

A kiss goodbye
A deep breath of fresh air
A tender hand squeeze to let you know they're
    right there
Homegrown tomatoes
Splashing in puddles
Feeling the raindrops trickle down your face
Your friend's laugh
Your dog who always knows when you're down
The cuddle with your nephew you've waited so
    long for
A cold ocean swim
The wild garlic you've picked
The loud buzzing of bees you thought was quiet
    until now
The community you didn't know existed
The smile from a stranger
The stars in the sky

The craving to enjoy the simple yet most meaning-
ful things life has to offer.
    For this I am so grateful.

I've loved, I've lost and I've healed. Yet all of it has felt so completely different from before.

I always thought I needed to win an Oscar, climb a mountain or travel the world to truly be successful. The past year has taught me that I could not have been more wrong. My success is within my relationships, my ability to see the joy in one fleeting moment and the lives I've touched with kindness. Society wants us to live bigger, buy more, to never be satisfied. Because there is no profit to be made from people who are happy with what they already have.

It is so true that being rich has nothing to do with money.

simplicity is beautiful.

– Rediscovering Gratitude –

August 2021

The tension in the theatre was the thickest it had ever been. I felt more sick with nerves than on our first preview show as we waited to hear the news we had all been dreading. Lights out. Venues across the country would be shutting their doors and going dark. For a whopping ten weeks! At the time it seemed unimaginable. The confusion in the Royal Shakespeare Company auditorium was palpable. Some actors burst into tears and others physically embraced for the last time in a while. The following day I cleared out my beloved dressing room while cast members disappeared off at staggered times to avoid contact and sad goodbyes. No wrap, no final bow and no emotional closure on what had been a joyful, dazzling run. To be robbed of the last lap left me feeling dispirited and bewildered.

As someone who has struggled with balance and the blues in the past, I tried to maintain a routine and to practise gratitude. It was important to take one day at a time. For me, that meant starting with a strong coffee by the River Avon every morning and repeating Rumi's words as a mantra, 'This too shall pass.' Totally scientific, of course it would pass – ideally within ten weeks! I looked for further inspiration. Harold Pinter regarded 'theatre as a serious business, one that makes or should make man more human, which is to say, less alone'. So with theatres shuttered, it begged the question, how to feel less alone, especially in isolation?

A coping mechanism came in the form of a jolting message from a colleague. A black screen with white block words imprinted boldly: 'Dear world, how does lockdown feel? Sincerely Gaza.' Curtails on freedom of movement, food shortages and curfews were new to us here. Perhaps these restraints might help us consider anyone under siege or those in the world suffering daily restrictions long before corona. This sobering thought made me realise my circumstances were certainly bearable. I would just need to find something to fill the void of theatre.

The desire to engage through technology was anything but burning. Perhaps the occasional meander through Google for more comforting quotes: 'Words are easy, like the wind...'. Easy for you to say, Shakespeare. We all know you wrote *King Lear* in quarantine during the plague. Or perhaps the more incentivising: 'We know what we are, but know not what we may be,' from *Hamlet*. Was quarantine, and all the subsequent sudden lockdowns, the moment to find out?

Growing up, I never felt I had a 'tribe' or community. Whilst I had supportive friends, I felt at odds with my place in the world. With different influences from Catholicism to Islam, and from Palestine to Ireland via a rather English boarding school, one thing was certain – I had an identity crisis. And with such an incongruous blend of seemingly incompatible cultures, was it any surprise? However, 2020 did offer me one welcome surprise. This new virtual world helped me seek out and discover other like-minded individuals. The more I spoke to artists with similar backgrounds, the more I realised we faced similar challenges and yearned for a network. I decided to create a theatre and film club for actors and writers of Middle Eastern heritage (or mixed like me!). We explore plays and films from different Arab countries or by the Arab diaspora and then discuss our responses to the various themes. This new found connection, friendship and solidarity reminded me of Equity's slogan, 'Stronger together', and it certainly felt that way ... even at a distance. And whilst a similar overworked phrase, 'We're all in this together', quickly became insufferable when absurd antics over loo rolls and packaged pasta proved otherwise, I started to understand the importance of community and meaningful conversations about shared mutual experiences.

Vanessa Redgrave once said, 'Theatre is as essential to civilisation as safe, pure water.' As a performer, this might seem like a self-important notion on which to ponder, but theatre can sooth the soul and stimulate the mind – it is therapy. Everyone can find solace and entertainment in the arts, from bankers bingeing box sets to community theatre in conflict zones. Whilst jokes and stereotypes might lead you to believe that actors are sensitive, vulnerable, highly-strung creatures (and occasionally I have found that to be true!), we are also well accustomed to uncertain times and the necessity for resilience in order to survive them.

The vast injustices suffered during that period remain unmeasurable, so it is important to acknowledge the mass devastation caused for so many people in so many ways. However, despite everything, there were some memorable moments of lightness and joy in 2020 and I know I am not the only one who found that strange period of stillness both healing and cathartic. And at times even farcical, like spotting an otherwise 'normal' looking gentleman wearing a Second World War gas mask in the queue for Waitrose.

Bizarre as it may be, this is the first time I feel I have reached true equilibrium; a sense of inner peace that I never thought possible in my life. Whilst I would never 'thank' lockdown, I am now thankful for what I have and for what I previously took for granted, with an even deeper appreciation for family, health and privileges like the roof over my head, the food on my plate and the shoes on my feet. Oh, and superfast broadband.

– Of the Old, Remembering –

She:
'I'll see you by the ice-house,'
Hand across her trembling lip, and left arm raised
    in the hated salute.
That night was the picture set off on a grotesque.

So the long watches of the sleepless night
    passed, and
She could feel her elegant declension
Suddenly loud, and died away.
February after February
She had to find her own way through his mouth
The half-tender effect of a pump in the
Incessant battle, against dirt, against, cold, came
    before her.

All that he believed, all that neither man was able
    to answer.
All except a dirty-faced little boy,
Happy to be present.
Their guns, and he.

She pictured herself.
Strange young woman.
Twice she lost her balance and fell off, giggling;
Clinging to a man she clearly did not love.

– Diary of a Junior Doctor During the Covid Crisis –

January 2021

This night shift has been one of the toughest of my four-and-a-quarter-year career as a junior doctor in the NHS. We are in the midst of the second wave of Covid-19 and the hospitals across London are taking an absolute beating. Ambulances are queueing up outside emergency departments, hospitals are suspending some non-emergency surgeries to increase facilities to manage Covid patients, and all the while some people on the internet somehow have the gall to maintain this is all a hoax. This is all too real, and it's getting worse.

The pandemic has presented me with difficult decisions more frequently. When do we decide that a patient is actually dying? How do we withdraw life-sustaining treatment in a humane and dignified way? What is the best way to discuss these decisions with patients and their families?

I am a GP trainee currently on a hospital-based placement, and tonight my responsibility is to look after patients already admitted to a medical ward.

Most of the night has been spent reviewing patients with likely or confirmed Covid-19, struggling to maintain blood oxygen levels and requiring supplementary oxygen to do so. Some are losing the fight and need additional help to breathe with mechanical ventilators on intensive care. Many are extremely sick and, sadly, two have already succumbed tonight.

At 5.00 am a nurse bleeps me about George, an eighty-three-year-old grandfather with chronic lung disease who I had personally admitted last night. He had classic symptoms of Covid – tiredness, muscle aches and loss of smell, as well as worsening shortness of breath, and had been looking really ropey. He had pleaded with me to get him home, to be reunited with his grandchildren, who, thanks to the pandemic, he hadn't seen for nearly a year. Things had looked bad yesterday and we were faced with an almost impossible choice: to keep fighting the good fight despite mounting discomfort, or to give him medication that would ease his distress but also reduce the respiratory drive that was helping to keep him alive. George was bright as a button but discussing this decision with him was complicated by the fact that he was wearing a noisy mask helping him to breathe, muffling his words. I could hardly hear him and had to ask him to repeat himself several times. He was adamant he wanted to fight. However, as he tired throughout the next day, he started accepting small doses of drugs to ease his suffering.

I call his nurse, who tells me that George had gone from bad to worse, and despite our best efforts, she now needs me to come to confirm his passing. It's hard news to hear and gut-wrenching to think how he had to die without any of his family there to comfort him. I think back to our initial conversation. Could I have been any clearer about his chances of survival? Could I have made his death any more comfortable? I still have several sick patients to see, so I push these thoughts to the back of my head. I will see George to confirm his death later.

When I eventually get time to verify his death, I have technically finished my shift and have handed over responsibilities to the day team. I examine him to confirm his death and am now faced with the unenviable task of informing his family. First, I phone his son. It is a terrible thing to tell someone their loved one has died, and not made any easier when you have to do it over the phone. I express my condolences and give him the number of the bereavement service, who will guide him through the process over the next few days.

Next, I have to tell George's wife. As it happens, she was admitted to hospital with Covid-19 the day after George. She is on the next-door ward and, although on oxygen, is breathing comfortably. Dressed from head to toe in PPE, I go to her bed and introduce myself. 'I'm afraid I have some bad news about your husband...'. I feel wretched as I break the news that she is now a widow. The rest of her family should be here, to hug her, to look after her, to mourn with her as she realises that her life partner is gone forever. As my shift is over and I have no further responsibilities, I have some time, and we sit in silence together for a while – I can think of no words that will help. How long can I stay to make it better? Ten minutes? One hour? Two? Eventually, I pass on the message from her son that he is thinking of her and sends his love, and would like her to phone him when she feels up to it. Again, I express my deepest condolences, and go. It is difficult to leave her, alone on a ward full of unwell strangers, with the constant hum of oxygen masks and the relentless, interminable beeping of various machines. This does not feel close to an ideal place in which to impart such devastating news.

I think about the next unfortunate soul who may be in a similar position to George. Will I do things any differently? Did we allow George to cling to the hope of survival too long, at the cost of more dignity and comfort in death? If we are more pessimistic about patients' chances of survival, how do we tell them? Luckily, these decisions are not purely mine to make. They are shared between patients, their families and medical professionals, and this is a comforting thought. Still, I resolve not to shy away from difficult conversations. We must understand that while we cannot always cure patients, we can give them something equally valuable: a calm, comfortable, peaceful death.

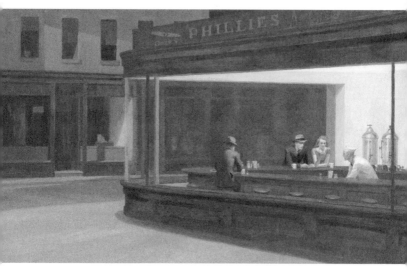

Nighthawks (1942) by Edward Hopper

– The Art of Being Alone Together | Edward Hopper's *Nighthawks* –

A floodlit diner glows green at a Lower Manhattan intersection. Like a fishbowl, its walls are curved and made of glass, giving us a good view of its starkly furnished interior: waxy lemon-yellow walls and a plain wooden door; a mahogany counter dotted with solitary salt and pepper shakers and lined with a row of vacant bar stools. Populating the diner at this brooding hour are four figures: a couple, a man drinking coffee and a uniformed employee. There's zero eye contact, zero conversation. They keep to themselves within this static bubble of time and space.

During lockdown, there was talk of all of us stay-at-homes trapped in an Edward Hopper painting. As we peered out of our living room windows; as we walked around an otherwise emptied block; as we perched on our beds and observed the eerie silence, a symptom of the dusty train tracks and missing planes overhead. In his deserted urban spaces and echoing landscapes, the twentieth-century American artist captures the sense of solitude that permeates modern life, pandemic or not. The beauty of *Nighthawks* – Hopper's best-known work, painted in January 1942, shortly after the United States had joined the Second World War – is that it shows we belong together even when we're apart.

Hopper's well-dressed couple are distinctly disconnected – he in his suit and tie, she in a crimson dress that matches her lipsticked mouth. He stares straight ahead with a smouldering look on his face and a skinny cigarette sandwiched between his fingers, while she fiddles with what looks like a folded dollar bill – time to pay? They're consumed by their thoughts, in different worlds, and yet their physical proximity and the symmetrical composition of their arms and hands bind them: their shoulders are comfortably hunched, their fingertips close. Though their features are stony, their body language is quietly tender, brushed with hope.

Judging by his appearance, the lone wolf on the near side of the counter could be an acquaintance of theirs. He, too, is snappily dressed: dark suit and steel-grey hat. However, he's by himself, a single white coffee cup by his elbow. There's something sinister about his presence at the centre point of the canvas, his back turned, unwilling or unable to look us in the eye, as if he has something to hide. Maybe he's just got off work. Or maybe he's skipped out early on drinks, he wanted some alone time – some alone time in the company of others. That includes the gaunt waiter who grimaces as he gets to work, the curve of his back testimony to his efforts. His shift isn't over, and these night owls are here to see it through with him.

Throughout the pandemic, hearing the gentle rumble of people clapping for the NHS on their doorsteps in the evening presented a sense of solidarity despite our ongoing solitude. Catching a glimpse of a child's rainbow taped to a cold plate-glass window raised the spirits and helped to maintain morale. We may have been distanced from one another – physically and emotionally – but once we knew when to listen and where to look, we no longer felt entirely alone.

Out on the street in *Nighthawks*, there's no sign of life, just a peculiar void of shadows. The inauspicious shopfront opposite is seemingly abandoned, as are the rooms glimpsed beyond the partially closed blinds. The fluorescent light is almost alien, and so is the muddied palette and that sickly shade of green. The artist had a keen interest in film and stage sets, which shines through in the painting's theatrical lighting. Outside looks decidedly less welcoming than inside.

Hopper's all-night diner is a refuge, a beacon in the dark. These uncommunicative souls may exist in emotionally isolated states, but at least they inhabit the same anonymous, transitory space. There's comfort in the mere proximity of others. We would know – shut out in the cold, looking in. An independent and somewhat elusive figurative painter, Hopper once described his works as an expression of his 'inner experience'. This is an inner experience to which we can all relate.

Spend some time with his rich and ambiguous art, and – like clouds after rain – your own feeling of isolation might start to lift. Aloneness is a theme in Hopper's moody painting, as it is in modern life. It will always be there, hiding in plain sight. The trick is to tackle it together – to find freedom in the blank space, relief in the silence. And you never know, perhaps behind the bar the distinctly disconnected couple's ankles are lovingly entwined. They're detached, and invisibly connected.

– *Extract from* A Book of Secrets –

Suffering

Never have we been better advised to be suspicious of the prioritising of convenience. It can misfire so badly when it is born from a desire to hook us to a product rather than a sensitivity towards our needs. It carries in its Shadow a damaging friction crueller than the one it seeks to destroy. When we are not bumping up against incompatible or abrasive information, we are not learning. We are neither growing nor becoming strong. Unpalatable information teaches us something about the ambiguity of the world; in the same way that those areas where we clash with our partners are commonly the fertile soil where we ourselves need to grow.

How might we, as inheritors of our Western mode (and unsure how comfortably we sit with that of Ancient China), face the frictions and disturbances of the world? Some young people, for example, now presume themselves to be delicate and even in physical danger when challenged by the friction of inconvenient ideas. And such delicacy has a habit of assuming authority, in the same way that the less secure partner in a relationship tends to be the more controlling, as the other learns to tread carefully and cater to prickly sensitivities. The Stoics, by means of contrast, taught us the fortitude that comes from only looking to control our own thoughts and actions – the only things we *can* control – and choosing to live peacefully with whatever else befalls us. The mistake, they suggest, is to try to manage things we cannot, which guarantees frustration and the sense of disturbance they were keen to circumnavigate. Sage advice from a people who knew of warfare and terror. *You are not fragile, you have all the resources you need,* they would say; and *it is not the world's responsibility to protect you, it can only be your own.**

---

* Before we roll our eyes at a bafflingly delicate younger generation, we might take a moment to recall our own responsibility. We did our best, but many of us, steeped in a culture saturated with therapies and self-help, protected our children from ever experiencing failure. As a generation, we ensured everything was defined as success, guaranteeing passes and awards for all; we may well have disproportionately helped with school work and over-managed their friendships and formative years. We largely denied them the opportunity to learn resilience. In effect, our own worries became a breeding ground for poor coping skills, a sense of entitlement, and a deeply anxious generation (who would go on to discover social media). But then, wait – were we not ourselves the offspring of parents who grew up in households darkened by the shadow of war, which enforced a leathery resilience at the expense of emotional subtlety? And so it continues, each new wave guided by fine intentions and broken compasses.

Without this Stoic wisdom, what is our default mode? We recreate what's familiar, we seek to control with little discrimination, and we distract ourselves with entertainment. To these ends we repeatedly find partners who create for us the same family dynamic we knew as children; we baulk and manipulate when they do not; we develop addictions and try to build futures that continually elude us; we binge.

These daily measures we put in place to ensure our world conforms to the story we prefer to tell about it, or to distract ourselves when it does not, are the familiar strains of being human. Remember Schopenhauer's diagonal line along which he plotted our life: the pull of our aims and strategical manoeuvres in one direction and that of blind Fortune in the other, correcting the gradient. The undulating line that climbs and dips along its x=y diagonal will bring us to an occasional peak: a great new job, a kind and beautiful new partner, a vibrant lucky streak in the face of life. And it appears in those moments that our strategizing and goal-planning have royally paid off, and while we modestly deflect praise, we inwardly congratulate ourselves on our magnificence. And then, on cue, Fortune reveals her hand. A lump on a loved one has leaked evil to her lymph-nodes; your phone has been stolen. In obvious and subtle ways, we are let down and our plans vanquished.

The Greeks knew it: life is tragic in its very structure. The *hubris* or pride that causes us to overreach ourselves will only invite the humbling response of Fate. Likewise, the Buddhists saw life as *dukkha,* which is often translated as 'suffering', but also incorporates a sense of impermanence and inevitable change. The Christian tale of life's suffering is inherited from St Augustine, who articulated to our collective unconscious the notion of Original Sin. They must be on to something.

Now let's sit with that for a moment. Sit in its *friction*. None of these schools of thought is telling us to despair. Each reminds us of our profoundly flawed nature in order to point towards a transcendental solution that might release us from its grip. We may not be especially attracted to the teachings of Buddha, or Christ, or know much about the Ancient Greeks, and so their particular answers might elude us. But a truth has been articulated for thousands of years, and with it a moving note of hope.

Despite all our attempts to distract ourselves, despite how frictionless we have grown to expect our world to be and how predictably we imagine our futures will fall into place if we plan well enough, a gravitational inevitability still drags us towards a centre that is difficult and heavy. We feel its centripetal pull not just at times of crushing tragedy, but also in the mundane moments of immovable sadness, when we are unable to sleep, gorged on Netflix, next to our partners and profoundly alone; or when we hover late in the evening by the living-room light switch, and a faint nausea stirs us as we notice our chairs and cups and objects are still arranged dumbly as we last left them, and will be so tomorrow.

We feel it in the ache of sadness yielded by love. A romantic relationship, once we are properly enveloped within it, has an undercurrent of tragedy. The note of despondency sounds as we realize every day that we are a disappointment to our partner; that they are too in return; that they are crueller to us than anyone else, and we to them; that our friends are kinder and seem to understand us better; that an active sexual life is no longer promised for the future; that we may not be desired; that something has silently left the room and will not return.

I am asked a lot, out here in New York, how it feels to be doing a Broadway run. The required answer is to describe perpetual and uncontaminated excitement. And it has been huge fun. New York sparks and fizzes with a galvanic charge, and at rare moments, performing a Broadway show seems to take that voltage and place it in my hands, streaking light between my fingers like the Tesla-gorged girls of those old Coney Island Electric Chair acts. Moreover, a tradition along the Great White Way decrees that famous actors and the like who are attending the show usually come round to say hello afterwards, and thus many nights have seen me frantically stuff socks into a drawer and greet the great and the good. At times this chimera of fluff and sparkle even resembles the self-aggrandising snippets and curated snapshots that comprise my social media feeds.

Sunday and Monday nights, however, offer no shows, and the sudden appearance of an early, empty evening in my production-provided apartment brings a baffling unpreparedness for the lack of company or excitement. They can be surprisingly, desperately lonely. In London, to decamp to my library for the evening with a book, a Scotch and a recalcitrant beagle-basset is a jealously protected treat I secure with stealth and guile, ushering my partner from the house with encouragements to see the world and explore. Now, I'm dogless in a white-walled flat, thousands of miles from home, and I haven't charged my Kindle. I've forgotten to make plans, it's too late to do work, and a first-night gift of dark Japanese whisky is looming from the side table, hinting at unsettling prospects. I don't even have the company of a partner from whom I can have the pleasure of separating myself.

Three months into a run and it's of course natural to pine for home. In my afternoon coffee-shop, writing in a busy, creamy world of frothing milk, frolicking babies and mashed avocado, I cannot locate the strange sadness I know will return if I don't plan for these shadowy, showless evenings. I put it down to missing my man, whom I cannot call in those dark times as he'll be curled up asleep in our big London bed, his head plopped off the pillow like a babbie. But I am more disturbed by the suspicion that I am suffering from a disappointment in being left truly alone with myself, which has rarely unsettled me in the past.

None of this is a tragedy, and it would be perverse to expect sympathy *(oh, does your provided New York apartment only have white walls? It sounds like a nightmare)*. But I am struck by how the fun of my time out here is conjoined to its assured reverse, and how impactful is the sudden absence of distraction. Distraction is the dazzling circumference of the circle: for me, it is performing the show, book-writing, *The Crown,* occasional dinners and drinks, sometimes buying clothes, days taken up with PR work. It is drawn wide around that dark centre whose pull I discern when none of the above is available and even the pale prospect of a blue-glowing e-Reader only accentuates a crushing, lonely failure of a night.

When the evening is like this, how comfortably isolation seems to fit us. How snug the sadness, how well tailored our particular worthlessness. We yearn for connection more than further distraction; the thought of watching another episode, or a fresh round of checking phone apps, only darkens the mood more. At least if we're in our home country we can scroll and flick through our contacts wondering who might be around, who might offer a glimmer of hope, which of our old cohorts' company will be less distressing than our loneliness, as if it were possible to summon the effort actually to go out and meet anyone.

You and I are then turned to that lumbering giant which accompanies us at all times: *our private life,* which leers back, embodying all our embarrassing, cheap, clumsy truths and shines disappointing daylight on our mysteries. Unable to summon even the energy to sit and read, now that all objects in the room have withdrawn and return only a mocking acknowledgement of their over-familiarity, I descend into a kind of blank stare, which provides at once the warmth of settling into the bosom of *something,* and at the same time, as I view myself from without, a horror at my inertia.

But it is here at this central, seemingly starless spot, I think, that we might identify a profound and surprising consolation.

The centripetal point

Our moments of misery, whether unexpected catastrophes or twilight intimations of the tragic structure of our biography, reveal to us the precise *weight* of life. The stubborn friction we feel as we cannot create the world we want, the sense of grinding halt as we stare into space and our eyes moisten for no reason our adult selves can discern: these moments reveal the true poundage of existence. And as we face our silent giant, it is almost impossible to imagine that we are now at the centre of things, that we now feel the true heft and business of life, that despite our desire for nothing but a return to bed, we might actually be *most alive.* Alive, that is, in the sickly, fearful distaste we feel for ourselves, which has seeped into the fabric and contours of our living room and now uncolours the scene, reducing our busy world of things to a membrane draped over drabness. But it is precisely there that we might catch a glimpse of life without distraction. Which means, *it is universal.* We are, at those moments, most profoundly connected to those from whom we feel inconsolably removed.

If we take a feeling of personal sadness and nudge it into a more charitable acknowledgement of the universal, we transform it into *melancholy.* Melancholy leans into the tragedy of life, but refuses to render misfortune our private property, or ourselves blameworthy. It allows our capacity for unhappiness, the fall-out of Fortune's inevitable friction, to find its resting place without destroying us. The alternative would be an inward-directed sadness, which takes a healthy regret for our beleaguered place in the world and muddies it with a conviction of personal failure. Melancholy does not try to resist the sadness, in fact it deeply feels its appropriateness, but it kindly directs our awareness out into a world teeming with fellow creatures each of whom, irrespective of outward success, face their private dark moments and are stalked by their own lurching monsters.

When we *personalize* our sadness, we may have fallen for the primrose promises of the snake-oil industry, and started to believe that through a lack of foresight, planning and self-mastery, we must be responsible for our failures. A grinning culture that assures us we can force fate into submission by personal effort will always point us to an equally personal failure when it inevitably reneges on its slippery pledges. At that point, like the faith-healer, it shrugs, proclaims it has nothing else to offer us, and blames our lack of faith. Naturally, a veil descends, and we suffer in silence. Our pain itself becomes a secret, because its roots connect it to a private place. Healthy melancholy may not fully cheer us up, but it extracts much of the poison.

The loneliness and tragic nature of romantic relationships, the fact that we are to be forever misunderstood and hectored by the person we are choosing to spend our life with – this too is transformed into common property, the correct weight of love. Viewed as an inevitable symptom of our common lot, we see it is neither our unworthiness nor our terrible misjudgement that has led to this impossible situation: it is merely the nature of two beings engaged in the implausible task of sharing their lives with each other. Good humour and self-forgiveness may turn out to be a better response than a continuous suspicion that you should be with someone else. The incessant hyper-sensitivity and bickering might mean that love is properly and appropriately in place. It may be difficult precisely for the reason that it is there to slowly and somewhat painfully transform us into better versions of ourselves.

Something magical happens when we reposition our perspective in this way. Unlike mere sorrow, melancholy does not seek to devour itself but instead it reaches out – it *yearns*. In this yearning (and the best melancholy music provokes this most clearly), desire, unknown when in the grip of depression, is reignited. When we acknowledge life's inevitable periods of tragedy and invite the consolation of commonality, the sense of our suffering stretches wide across the surface of the planet, through the hearts of those who brush past us on rainy streets, those whom we see alone through a window, and those who live and endure on the other side of the world.

It pushes too at the edges of our comprehension: we might vaguely acknowledge that we all share in pain, but the image of quite what that means, extended across so many people and back and forth across time, is a far harder image to contain. In losing something of the specificity of our selves into the generality of the human, we are moving into the queasy realm of the boundless. At this point we can emerge from the dense woods and meet with an expansive and surprising panorama: that of the ancient Sublime.

– On the Tenth Anniversary of Patrick Leigh Fermor's Death or 'Twas Me What Done 'im In ... –

I am afraid that, just as Eliza Doolittle might have said of gin in *My Fair Lady*, so of Paddy Leigh Fermor I could remark, 'I think it was me what done 'im in.'

I never met Paddy, but not for want of trying on either side; ours was a unique relationship of rooms-just-left, right-weeks yet wrong-countries, if-only-we-had-knowns or you-should-have-saids, filled instead with lengthy exchanges, a constant correspondence often with erroneous enclosures like hearing aid invoices and extended conversations on the telephone between Kardamyli and Dorset that lasted for hours as he very kindly agreed to edit much of my first book, *In the Dolphin's Wake*; the tale of my five-and-a-half-thousand-mile journey through the Greek islands from Venice to Istanbul in 2006. I still have the pencil marked papers – 'de trop' being a favourite comment.

Four years and twenty-seven rejections later, my courageous newly appointed publisher,

Anthony Weldon, at Bene Factum, came up with the outlandish suggestion that Paddy might actually endorse my work. A scheme so fraught with eventuality that Elpida Beloyannis, Paddy's devoted housekeeper, was driven to the point of near nervous breakdown and the diminutive publishing house to its knees, thanks to exorbitant courier charges alone.

'e love your book very much, Harry, but every time he put it down, he can't remember where he left it,' an exasperated Elpida explained to me over the phone long distance from the Mani. Indeed, towards the end, so great were the number of printed manuscripts sent out to Kardamyli, there was one in every room of the house and almost one on every side table too. 'Your bloody book, 'i's everywhere,' the beleaguered retainer would cry.

But as the days wore on, so the possible seemed to grow ever impossible and, just weeks before Paddy's death, we were told to prepare a quote which he would sign off – reluctantly we agreed and my redoubtable editor, Alan Ogden, manfully squared up to the unenviable task of drafting something 'in the style of' which the more we tinkered with, grew ever more unremarkable, contrived and least Fermoresque. Hastily despatched to Athens, either the gods were smiling, I was up to date with Her

Majesty's Revenue & Customs, or both, I shall never know, but almost by return an envelope arrived in Paddy's unmistakable if shaken hand – it contained two printer labels with kind words that *only* he could have written and *only* I could have dreamed of.

The truth of the matter is, I suspect, In the *Dolphin's Wake* was quite possibly the last thing Paddy ever read – hence my, perhaps now, not so outlandish opening statement.

But Paddy was very kind and generous to me, which he needn't have been, and yet he was, despite being desperately ill in his last year; rare traits these days. But these are gifts which define him as a special and unique character in my life, whose wholly undeserved words make him stand out not just for the past but for the future as well.

We launched *Dolphin* in the Officers' Mess at Wellington Barracks on 9 June 2011; the same day Paddy flew back to England for the last time. As I mentioned his name in my speech, not only did a great cheer go up from the assembled guests but the massed bands of the Guards Division, preparing to beat the retreat, broke into fanfare on the drill square below and an enormous rainbow appeared in the sky behind me; folk will scoff, and rightly so, but, at the time, it was as if he was patting me on the back and urging me on.

We partied till dawn and, later, walking home, I rang Elpida to report how things had gone the night before. It was then she told me that Paddy had died.

You will appreciate therefore that, alas, mine is but a pitiful walk-on part at curtain, already lost in a crowd scene – I have no *cause célèbre* claim to Paddy's memory other than, some might argue, that my beginning started with Paddy's end. Not the greatest of accolades and it has certainly been a steady yet raucous downhill ever since, as many will no doubt happily and freely testify, but nonetheless, Patrick Leigh Fermor stands like a lone figure in a landscape lost to time. Adventurer, war hero and writer, his deeds – the stuff of legends – lie testament to the memory of a great man, known to the Greek andartes as the immortal Philedem!

– Two Grains of Sand –

By noon the sandstorm had swallowed everything more than an arm's length away. Even the giant wind turbines, that just the night before had been blinking reassuringly-red on the horizon, were now lost, as though they had never existed. It was worse in the streets: they sucked up the sand and the wind and whipped them up to a terrible speed. Naturally, none of the residents of Tibansar had expected a sandstorm in January – it was not the season. Before they realised what was happening and managed to close the shutters, their living rooms were full of the powdery, brown sand of the Thar desert. Those too far away from their homes were forced to duck into the nearest shop, café or even a house that was willing to have them (most were, as sandstorms always seemed to produce an urgent sense of solidarity in Tibansar).

'The Venturi effect,' said the man with the moustache, looking out of the window, as the sand pressed in waves against the ancient, yellow façades with their intricate engravings of shells, tigers, deities.

It took a moment for Dirk to catch on that the man was addressing him.

'I'm sorry?'

'The Venturi effect,' he repeated, speaking with a slight accent – Dutch, maybe.

'Ummm,' nodded Dirk, as though he had understood, and returned to his book, but was presently interrupted again when the front door burst open. For a few seconds the silence of the bookshop ceded to a howling whistle as a young woman fought against the wind, pressing her back against the door to force it shut.

The shop owner ran over to help, his sandals slapping sharply against his heels, and shouting, 'Goodness me!' over and over. When they succeeded, it was as if the air had been sucked out of the room. The fluttering curtains and napkins, whirling about without intent, suddenly froze and fell.

She wiped her forehead, licked by strands of brown hair, and brushed her forearms ineffectively.

'Are you alright, miss?' asked the gentle, round-faced owner.

To Dirk's surprise the woman replied in Hindi, quickly and naturally.

'Please,' said the owner with a vague gesture, inviting her to sit down. The woman asked for a coffee and surveyed the bookshelves first. A little pool of sand formed around her as she did so, fed by thin cascades from her hair and clothing. She picked a large volume and sat down at the opposite end of Dirk's table (it was a very cramped shop).

She must have seen him looking because she asked – rather offhandedly, in a way one speaks to a guest that's been neglected all evening: 'Have you come across this before?'

'Yes ... no, I mean. I haven't. But I've heard he's very good,' replied Dirk. The question had caught him unawares; he didn't realise he had been hoping for one.

'I love his style. It's very hard to make ... thank you ...,' she took the coffee, '... make biography readable.'

To Dirk's surprise she opened the book halfway and started reading from a random passage. He returned to his own book too, though it felt silly in comparison: a frivolous novel, set on an entirely different continent. His body was in India and his mind elsewhere. 'I may as well not be here at all,' he thought and put it down.

'I can vouch for her, however,' he said, pointing to a novel above the woman's head. This was a lie of sorts. Though he owned the book, he had never read it.

'Really? Good? Well, why not then...,' she

handed the copy over to the shop owner. 'What?' she asked on seeing Dirk's puzzled expression.

'Just like that?' he said laughing.

'Why not? You recommended it.' She seemed in all earnestness surprised.

'Yes, I suppose.'

'Don't worry, even if it's no good. I've run out of books already and it's best to stock up.'

'That's a wonderful problem to have,' said Dirk. 'I'm almost there, too. Unfortunately most of the stuff I brought with me, I didn't like very much.'

'That's a pity. And where have you been?'

'The North mainly. I've made quite a long stopover here, though – longer than I expected. Strangely, I like it a lot.'

'Have you been to the desert?' she asked. The hint in her voice was unequivocal – people came to Tibansar for the desert, not the town.

'Yes, but it was very unadventurous. They just took us to a sand dune on the border and cooked us some dahl. I've never felt more like a tourist. God, and that camel ride.'

'Tourist!', she sneered. 'There's nothing more touristy than this town.'

'Which is why I love it! It feels like a bad movie set. But it's undeniably historic. And after all the suffocating cities.'

'You've not enjoyed yourself then?'

'Well...' Dirk felt under scrutiny all of a sudden. 'How long have you been travelling? To have churned through all your reading, that is.'

The window frames groaned under the weight of the wind, though it had subsided somewhat.

'Oh, no, I'm not travelling. I live in Gujarat. I'm just here for a few days.'

'Gujarat?'

'Does that shock you?' she asked, knowing well that it did.

'Not shock, not exactly. You just don't – errr – don't normally meet young Western women living in a place like Gujarat. You're ... American?'

'No,' she gave a rakish smile. A one-zero smile. 'Canadian. I'm Audrey, by the way.'

'Dirk!'

They shook hands across the table and Audrey explained her peculiar situation: she was a student from Winnipeg but was spending a year in a village in rural Gujarat, documenting the effects of a nearby coal-fired electricity plant. Besides monopolising and underpaying the local workforce, the plant had destroyed the surrounding land, in more ways than one. The pollution had brought about acid rain, damaging the harvests. The rivers, she said, and even the entire Bay of Gujarat, were completely dead – no wildlife could survive in waters that were systematically treated as a dumping ground. And all of this was happening in broad daylight, with the full complicity of the state, as the plant's owners were too rich and well connected to be punished.

They both ordered another coffee. The man with the moustache had fallen asleep, his book still open.

'It's infuriating what these people have done to the local villages in – what? the space of three years? Every man is either being worked to the bone or has had his livelihood destroyed. And now they're all drinking to cope with it. And beating the women, too. Domestic abuse is through the roof.'

'I thought Gujarat was a dry state.'

'It is. They cross the border and drive it back, or brew it at home. It's a harsh penalty if they get caught... I know a man who had his hand chopped off by the village elder.'

'Surely not...'

'You'd be surprised. It's not legal justice, of course. The elder ended up in prison.'

Audrey gave a short, serrated laugh, like a faulty chord, but presently covered her mouth. 'I'm sorry,' she said, shaking her head. 'I've reached a bit of a strange impasse. Besides, even if my work is published, it won't make a difference.'

Dirk felt indignant – why, or whether on her behalf, he couldn't say. 'And you find that funny?'

'Oh no. I was laughing more at how quickly I've become accustomed to my village. No electricity – the irony, right? No electricity, no running water, barely a bed. And I'm totally fine with it. In fact, I'm not sure how I'll get used to Winnipeg again.'

'What do you do all day when you're not working? Do you have any colleagues with you?'

'Yes, there's a French girl with me from Bordeaux, but we don't get along very well.'

Dirk was listening intently, resting his head in one hand.

'When there's really nothing to do,' she continued, 'I take bangh and listen to music. That's actually why I came here. Tibansar is the nearest place you can get it.'

'Bangh?'

'Come on!'

'No, really.'

'It's like marijuana, but "the male version" of the plant.'

'Is it legal?'

'Sure. You can buy it here.'

Dirk shuffled in his seat. They had been sitting like so for a while and his legs were starting to hurt. The shop owner's brother – grinning, clearly delighted to have customers despite the weather – took away their coffee cups.

'My bus goes this evening but I can show you later in the afternoon. It's just outside the city walls,' she said.

'If it's not any trouble.'

In the end it did turn out to be trouble: it was some time before the storm subsided and Audrey's bus was now due to leave in an hour. However, she still insisted on accompanying Dirk to the bangh dealer.

Having settled the bill, and Audrey paid for her books – which she carried tucked under her arm, schoolgirl-wise – they made their way through the meandering alleyways to the main square and out to the Old Town's great, wooden gateway.

The heat had picked up with a ferocity that, like the sandstorm, was unheard of in January – as if trying to make up for its earlier absence – and some of the bonhomie between Dirk and Audrey evaporated in the blistering sun. The rubbish bags out on the streets had been ripped up by stray dogs and now festered and stunk. Bikers – mainly on knock-off Enfields – charged through with little care for themselves or the pedestrians.

'You're right. I've changed my mind,' said Audrey,

catching up with Dirk, who as a habit always walked too fast. 'The scooters are the worst thing about the country. Have you been to Mumbai? It's wonderful in Mumbai – in part because they don't have...'. Dirk couldn't make out the rest: it was lost in the roar of a Triumph, carrying a four-person family, that nearly ran over his foot.

'Christ!' he shouted as the motorbike whistled past.

Crowds jostled around the shops and on street corners. Most people seemed to be outside simply for the sake of it. Passing down the long, cobbled thoroughfare that linked the Jain temples with the main square, Dirk waved to a friend of his, a miniaturist whom he had met the week before, as they walked past his shop, which was as small as the works he produced.

'He writes little poems on scrap paper,' said Dirk over his shoulder, hitching up his backpack.

'Who?'

'That man we just passed. Kamal. He's a painter – not a very good one – but a brilliant poet. At least I think so. He writes little poems on scrap paper every day and then throws it out of his balcony window. Whoever reads it, reads it.'

'That's –'

'Beautiful, isn't it?'

'I was going to say littering.'

On the main square, cries of various rupee values, all more or less trivial, rose into the air as salesmen advertised coconut water and dosa. Their stalls were three-deep with people all waving flimsy banknotes. Opposite them, under the shade of the Rajput's palace, stood a large group of tourists, confused and immobile like a lost herd.

Dirk noted that Audrey's neck, still covered in sand, was going red. He gave a smile, which she half-returned. 'Sure you don't want to put your books in my bag?'

She looked around and squinted. 'No, that's alright.'

'Ok, lead the way.'

They said little during the steep descent to the town gate, where any hint of historic charm came to an abrupt end, where poorly tarmacked reality and the suburbs began. This deflating transition was not helped by the rickshaw drivers, who pounced on Dirk and Audrey's fair, foreign appearance. Even her Hindi was of no use: most of the drivers didn't understand it, as the dialect spoken in these parts was Marwari, and those who did, bewildered by the novelty, called their friends to come see the *firangi* that spoke Hindi.

'It's just here,' said Audrey in an exasperated tone. She ushered them into a courtyard. The bangh shop was at the far end, behind a see-through plastic curtain. Dirk couldn't help but picture a cross between a butcher's and a strip club: there was a curiously squalid, unpleasant undercurrent to the place. Inside, in a pint-sized room painted red, a young couple, evidently backpackers, drifted in and out of consciousness, two empty milkshake glasses on the table in front of them, while a fat Indian man kept watch. He was sitting on a tiny stool that was far too small for him, so that it looked like three wooden sticks were sticking out of his ass.

Audrey said something and the man gave her a tattered menu that Dirk scanned over her shoulder without taking anything in.

'They've had quite a dose,' she said, looking at the couple. The girl was drooling slightly out of the corner of her mouth. Her hand, unnaturally twisted under her back, made Dirk feel nauseous. He looked at his watch.

'How many do you want?' Audrey asked.

'There's a quantity?'

'Sorry, I didn't explain – cookies are best. They last longer. You can buy them in packs of five.'

'Five, then.'

A quick exchange followed between Audrey and the fat man, who produced two brown-paper packages.

'Don't mix with alcohol', he says. She nodded in thanks. 'I got you ten. It's 1,200 rupees.'

That had been the last of Dirk's cash. All he wanted to do now was head back to the hotel and stand under a cold shower, but he walked Audrey back to the main square first, where her bus was due in ten minutes. They stood on the cobbles in silence, their eyes scanning the square with forensic preoccupation. The crowd felt more oppressive somehow, although it had thinned out. Families sat on top of enormous suitcases, the women wearing brilliant sarees, the children almost nothing, and Dirk wanted to say something or at least offer his thanks again for showing him the bangh shop, but all he could focus on was the golden-orange light as it caught the balconies of the Rajput's palace. He didn't want the cookies at all. He didn't know why he had bought them, and would probably put them in the bin as soon as he got back to his room.

– Growing Pains –
Spring 2020

I've waited a long time for this. Ten long years of urban prowling, and finally I find myself in lockdown liberation with a garden the size of Green Park. Happily, my partner-in-crime is horticulturally competent, keen with a trowel and happy to share his garden haven with me.

Now, I really *mustn't* get too over-excited.

This is a brave new world for gardening newbies. The possibilities are endless, but we are faced with the sudden impossibility of sourcing seeds we now simply *cannot* live without. Thank God for the bartering system that flourishes out of nowhere, and what a way to share our adventure with friends. We start trading sausages for seeds, fresh bread for beans and eggs for their cartons. Asking a lot of stupid questions, we begin to piece together what we need to do, and what *we absolutely mustn't do*.

The sun shines and we pot in contentment. Containers are plucked from obscurity at the back of the cupboard. We dash in soil, study the envelopes carefully and drop in the tiny specks, wrinkly nuggets, shiny beads. Shimmy on some compost. Push down gently. Label with a sharpie. Lacking a greenhouse, we test each windowsill for the hottest and voila! The indoor hothouse is born.

I water with reckless abandon then realise that the seeds are drowning. Queue mild panic – am I now a seedling murderer? Each morning I pad downstairs, armed with my usual green tea, and bend over the brown mulch forest of eggcup cartons, takeaway boxes, and plastic trays. Despite my best stares, nothing stirs. Patience is not my bedfellow. Perhaps just a *dash* more water?

Days passed. Heading outside, the old veggie garden is attacked with gusto and before long, and rather miraculously given that garden centres are still shut, we have fully functioning raised beds. We clink mugs and toast our success. Later, the dog is discovered having an afternoon nap on the warm soil. We fear our reprimands fall on deaf ears.

There is great debate about where to plant the artichoke, gifted by a dear friend. Finally we choose a cosy spot by the beloved echium. Not a week has passed before the slugs move in on its floppy ears, and it now resembles a cheese plant. Thus the first hard lesson of gardening is learnt – eyes off the prize at your peril. The artichoke is added to the morning roster of visits and I become eagle-eyed to slimy trails, catapulting each culprit across the lawn. Eggshells now dry in the kitchen, ready to be crushed and sprinkled.

It is a dwarf pea that provides me with a first peek at its lime-green shoot, greeting me a hearty good morning and a how-do-you-do. I cannot deny a squeak of excitement. More green arrives and the egg boxes brim over. I am a proud mother hen. The French beans bound up in a matter of days. Another tray now contains what looks like grass but will apparently become leeks. As instructed, I dutifully tickle each seedling, having sternly informed my partner-in-crime that this trick is *not* an old wives' tale. Friends ask after my 'plant babies'. Oh dear, I think I *might* be broody.

I swot up on techniques, informing and confusing myself in equal measures. Before long we are traipsing across the garden weighed down by trays of little victories, each a hopeful offering to the spring sunshine. Soon the peas are out and thriving, the potatoes snug in their sleepy ditches. The onions look a bit bedraggled and our broad beans are floppy, but we are proud as punch. We wait hopefully for the 'last frost in May'. I don't know when this will be, but I am hoping one of my gardening friends will let me know when it has passed.

Our fears are realised when we find the dog

sunbathing on top of the potato beds again. Lines of defence are constructed out of canes and stern looks. The dog replies mournfully. Despite his best efforts, within days we count three, four, five shoots through the soil. We 'earth up', and back to sleep the potatoes go. A little later we eat our first haul of lettuce. Neither of us comment on its slight bitterness, delighted as we are to have grown even the most unpalatable of produce.

Whilst in my working life I am used to words doing what I tell them, the garden is not quite like that. Sometimes nature has other plans for you. I am heartened by the successes and confused by the non-starters. We battle the wind, slugs, and seeds that simply refuse to germinate, despite our best stares *and* the correct amount of water.

Having gone from nought to sixty in the space of two months, I now can't imagine a life un-governed by the seasons, growing in knowledge year-on-year, clinking our mugs over each little triumph, our faces bronzed and boots muddy. Just like that, we are gardeners, reconnecting with 'the good life' that was waiting for us all along.

MARK CORETH

– Reflections on Flight –

If I were told that my time was up, life had been lived and now I should shuffle on to the unknown, I would be a little sad and I would plead for a bit more. There is still far too much to try to achieve, too much that I long to witness before I place my last full stop. Equally, however, I would have to thank the Lord for giving me so many opportunities, so many balls to catch and run with. Life is a book filled with a series of chapters across the spectrum of drama, challenge and emotion. I feel that I have been blessed with a life that has been centred around a happy and fulfilling family, adventures and careers that have so suited me. If I am to open that book at one chapter, I think it would be this: 'FLIGHT', as I feel that in so many ways it sums up the book as a whole in hope, aspirations and appreciations.

As a child, I remember getting a copy of Richard Bach's book, *A Gift of Wings*, which is a series of short stories and reminiscences of people, planes, of flying and of the freedom of flight. Bach is the author of numerous books. Most notably, and I suspect best known, is his short story, *Jonathan Livingston Seagull.* He is also a hugely experienced pilot, from the fast jet to barnstorming across the United States in old biplanes. His books remain always beside my bed. I am far short of Bach in my experiences in the air and in the types flown; indeed I am a beginner to so many a pilot. The real magic of flight, however, is not what other people do, but is what you yourself do, your experiences and your spirit of adventure. Flight is very personal. I have 1,700 odd hours in my log book, the majority of which were flown over the past ten years in just one aeroplane, a Jodel D1051 Special, and to me she is a most special machine – made of wood and canvas, minimal instrumentation, flight by the seat of your pants and not fast. G-AYLC, as she is registered, has given me a taster of Richard Bach's religion of flight.

The experience of flight takes a number of forms. A short flight amongst fair weather cumulus, a dusk landing, the practice of all that can happen, meant or unmeant. One of the greatest pleasures is introducing flight to others, young and old, seeing and feeling their elation running wild. Flight is always about learning, improving and usually pushing your boundaries that little bit further. The pilot who flies the circuit of his local airfield will one day want to land elsewhere. That elsewhere, with a leap of faith, may be across the English Channel to France and then one day maybe to Belgium, to Germany and beyond. My first flight to France was in a small single seat biplane, G-BXMX, my Currie Wot. It was a flight with every bit as much challenge and excitement as my first solo. We then flew on to a wedding party in Bremgarten, Germany, my boundaries truly stretched, crossing mountainous terrain and huge stretches of forest. However, it was with G-AYLC that I really found my wings spreading wide both within the British Isles and beyond, sometimes shared and at other times solo.

It is easy enough to fly on a beautiful day around your home field, but flight over any distance can so often be a challenge, not least of all due to weather. High pressures and low pressures, weather fronts and winds, all add to excitement and challenge. Decisions must be made, to fly or not, to divert or not, and when far from home, the desire to return can blur the decisions you might make. Diversions into airfields unknown and unplanned will invariably reveal the hidden world of people and places that you would otherwise have overflown and missed out on. The more you fly, the more your limits are revealed to you and the more you can push them again that very little bit. Diversions need not be a fear or regret but a source of challenge and excitement. Take, for example, a flight that I made when, as a sculptor, I was casting a monumental dragon at a foundry in the Czech Republic. I had flown to the fine and friendly airfield in the local town of Vrchlabi in the mountains to the north of Prague. I needed to inspect the sculpture before it was to head off to Saint-Emilion in the Bordeaux region of France, for installation just two days later. My route should have taken me southwest over Bavaria abeam Switzerland and into France but there was an impenetrable slow moving weather front that stretched from the Alps right through to the coast of Holland. To fly my little aeroplane through it was not an option. Taking a commercial flight was, but equally it would have felt like defeat. My Jodel and I therefore rerouted, flying past Dresden, a city steeped in history and so nearly bombed to total destruction towards the end of the Second World War. We flew on past Paderborn, where I was once based with my regiment. On we flew, over the Möhne Dam, destroyed during the infamous Dambusters raid on the night of 16–17 May 1943. We landed in deteriorating weather at Hilversum in Holland, before hooking behind the weakening front and routing down the coast to Normandy and Bordeaux in time for the dragon's installation. That was success; it was elation in outrunning the gremlins that were trying so hard to obstruct my plans. There is a saying that you should never mix business with light aviation. True ... but equally there is a little bit of devil in all of us.

The magic of a small aeroplane is in the freedom that it gives you, the freedom to fly through air once occupied by aerial warriors and indeed to look down upon the horrors that were the frontlines of recent history. Flying over Flanders you see cemeteries stretching beyond both wing tips ... you feel the terror of the trenches below and the crack of the bullets from the ghosts of aerial combat. G-AYLC has carried me to the battlefields of Balaclava, the Crimea, en route visiting the catastrophic horrors of Auschwitz. We flew to the Crimea just months before it was annexed by Russia. That airspace is now largely contested; it is a war zone. Instead, your route might be taking you more peacefully past Innsbruck through the staggering beauty of clear alpine air for a landing at Zell Am See, high in the mountains, but far below their snow-covered peaks. Flying on through Pass Lueg, with rocks at your wing tip and Hitler's Eagle's Nest above, the juxtaposition between beauty and the chill of history. Just ten minutes later you find yourself on the final approach to Salzburg International Airport and the city, one of Austria's jewels, with such close family ties that I feel almost at home.

I could go on and on describing flights that I have shared with my Jodel, sculpting trips to the Białowieża forest in Poland, the home of the European bison or down the Danube to the Carpathian Mountains in Romania, where bears were my subject. To Gibraltar, Majorca, the extraordinary island of Malta whose population was awarded the George Cross for valour during the Second World War. Every trip hands one the magic of flight, the accrued challenges of distance, be they thunderstorms or foreign airspace. Each trip awards you exhausted but satisfying nights in new places with new sights, sounds, foods and cold draughts of reviving beer. How happy it is when these experiences are shared by my passenger or other aeroplanes in company, yet there are times when flight can be best appreciated on your own, however selfish that may be ... private memories and private dreams.

In 2016, I was commissioned to make a sculpture for the Order of St John to be placed in Muristan in the heart of the most holy Old City of Jerusalem, a city that had always beckoned me. The work was to tell of the history of Jerusalem, her people and to give a message of hope for the region and the world beyond. I made a Tree of Hope, a bronze olive tree with its roots going into the heart of the city but exploding from its canopy were migrating swifts; the tree symbolising the walls of Jerusalem and the swifts symbolising the people. Beyond the tree I now have bronze swifts flying in formations of three around the world, my prayer flag that the Abrahamic faiths – all of whom have their roots in the city – may fly like pilgrims together. As an integral part of this sculpture I brought together Flight2Hope which took place on 2 April 2019. With seven other aeroplanes from the United Kingdom, we flew a stormy Mediterranean Sea to Eilat in the south of the Holy Land. With my Jodel in the lead and aeroplanes crewed in equal numbers by members of the Abrahamic faiths, men, women, boys, girls, professors, generals, motorbike mechanics and an astronaut, Fight2Hope flew up the Jordan Valley along the Dead Sea. Astonishing terrain, desert, mountains, a history of literally biblical proportions. We flew over to Amman in Jordan and then back around Jerusalem, with the migrating swifts whipping past our canopies. We crossed religious and political borders, we carved a message of hope and mutual respect in the air above the Holy Land with our aeroplanes, before then flying home and finding relief in a hugely successful and, I believe, important mission.

If there is one flight that will be held in my mind as the ultimate for me, it has to be Flight2Hope. Whatever follows will be merely a bonus, even if it were to be a world tour. If this flight had been my full stop, I know I could and would have saluted and hung up my goggles and helmet with a feeling of gratitude for a happy and fulfilling chapter.

Yes, it is tempting to ask, hope or even expect more, be that within this chapter of flight or indeed in the book as a whole, and so ask for more, with some humility, I certainly shall. Please, dear Guardian Angel, may I fly for as long as Air Commodore 'Daddy' Probyn did. Probyn was a remarkable balloon-busting pilot of the First World War who eventually retired to Kenya. I remember meeting him when I was a child as he flew into Kilifi in his Jodel D9 Bebe, an aeroplane he built himself and in which he flew for twenty odd years over the East African bush. Daddy Probyn took his last flight on his ninetieth birthday, after which he hung up his goggles and donated the aeroplane to the Aero Club at Wilson Airport in Nairobi. He was a man in charge of his destiny. Little did I know as a young enthusiast watching him swing the propeller and trim the aeroplane with elastic bands stretched from the joystick to strategically placed hooks around the cockpit, that I, too, would fall so deeply for an aeroplane of the very same family, a Jodel. G-AYLC is a little bigger, she carries two people, she has more power and bigger fuel tanks, but in every other way is the plane built and flown by that remarkable man, Daddy Probyn.

My small request, please Guardian Angel, is that I too can hang up my goggles on my ninetieth birthday in 2049. G-AYLC will by then be eighty-four, we will have had forty years of flying together. 2049 – we have a good twenty-seven years of new adventuring ahead of us.

SUSIE CORETH

– A Journey Around My Bedroom –

February 2020 | A response to the 1794 book,
Voyage Autour de ma Chambre,
by Xavier de Maistre

I wake. It's six o'clock and dark as night,
The room is freezing cold, the fire long dead,
I could snooze the alarm; shall I? I might,
And stay curled in my temporary bed.
But something itches me to start my day,
I lift the duvet, shivering and stand
Lightheaded in the cold, my body sways,
Longing for a coffee in my hand.
This room is tiny: bed, kitchen and desk,
A fireplace, some shelving lined with books,
A place to eat, to sleep, to work, to rest,
A bedroom that becomes a writer's nook.
And now the taste of coffee fills the air
With warmth and brain fuel, so I start my day
In these, the silent hours; nothing there
To stop my mind and pen having their way.
I've always found these hours are the best,
Most fruitful, when my brain is most alive,
That's why I'm here, on this solo quest:

To give myself a final chance to thrive.
And thus, this bedroom changes hour on hour,
Evolving on my mind's perpetual whim,
To be whatever I need it; there's its power –
It stops me from sinking, lets me swim.
This tiny bedroom plays the crucial part:
As I journey round my mind, it holds my heart.

– Going Round in Circles –
August 2021

To avoid being overwhelmed by the tragedy and frustration of the pandemic, the mind turns gratefully towards trivial reflections. What appears, from diagrams and drawings, to be a round coronavirus, with little spikes sticking out all over, like a weapon hurled by a giant in a cartoon, has introduced a swirling morass of circles, of all sizes and dispositions, beginning of course with a zero. 'Nothing can come of nothing,' it has been said, but perhaps something can.

The most obvious circle to me at the moment is the symbol on the screen of my laptop, telling me that there is no wi-fi – for what reason, who knows. There is also the plethora of little round-faced fashionable dogs, bouncing along the pavements. Beyond that, the circle we hear most about is Earth, spinning hotly in the universe. We ourselves rotate between horror at the prospective bake-off and fascination at the science being demonstrated, and hope that human ingenuity will somehow squeeze us through the crisis. The other global feature is the pandemic, about which we have rather similar thoughts. 'Global' sounds more frightening and inevitable, but there have always been viruses everywhere; they reappear in cycles. This one seems to have brought all its relatives to the feast at the same time, and so it is our responsibility to make sure that the feast disagrees with them.

What is the virus like? How does it operate and
     why did it come?
Does it fly through the air with the greatest of ease?
Does it travel with animals, fungi or fleas?
Does it track us, relentless, on scooters and skate-oes
To drop on our heads like a sack of potatoes?

How to get away from it has exercised governments deeply since the pandemic started. The best answer would be vaccination, but at first it lay in the concept of isolation and the wearing of masks. With any luck, the masks would protect us from the entry of the virus – if the effect of masking did not make us unrecognisable – so that it would retreat in confusion. As for isolation, this unwanted condition had to be made more palatable by a pretty name for being locked up (or down) in a defined space, but where? Because cages are for canaries

coops are for chickens

cells are for anchorites

cupboards are for crockery

cabins need logs, and

closets are for coming out of.

So – the new identity of the bubble was revealed. Bubbles are for blowing, of course (but better not, as you might spread infection), but it was not a real bubble, because, however beautiful and flexible they are, such bubbles would be hopeless at protecting us from infection; we would use up the air in minutes and, breaking the bubble, would run into the virus, waiting outside to hamper our breathing as well. No, at the height of the emergency the idea was to be in your house or flat, alone or with a small number of the same people, with whom you would be 'bubbled' for what seemed like all eternity. If you had a garden, it was fine to exercise in it. If you did not, the apartment became your stamping ground, to the detriment of the carpet, although there was the thrilling expectation, once a week, of being able to take the rubbish out and walk a few yards down the road – and back.

As it happens, I have been 'bubbled' with King Edward VII and Queen Alexandra. This was not just because of writing Alexandra's biography, but also that two cut-out life-size figures, which were once used in an exhibition, are keeping me company. It could have been a lot worse: they are quiet and kindly, do not interrupt or require any kind of ministration, and do not contradict or argue if I throw the occasional remark in their direction. Their very presence shows the circular nature of my interests; having been 'introduced' to Queen Alexandra when I was about seven, she has appeared regularly ever since, especially during my working years, and now she has come back, not with a vengeance but with a flourish. She herself was aware of bubbles in the form of sparkling spa waters, which reminded her of foaming bottles of champagne.

Beyond the bubble, there is always the view out of the window and this depends largely on luck. In my case, the nearest approximation to a garden is the churchyard opposite, containing wonderfully massive and ancient trees. One, a huge chestnut, perhaps at least 200 years old, had developed a vast, curved dome, which, on the skyline, seemed to have little sprigs sticking out all round the edge. Just like the virus, I thought, and while this did not spoil my affection for the tree, neither did it increase my respect for Covid-19, although they were somehow linked. However, I am sorry to say that stormy weather made a big branch fall off, damaging a nearby building.

Like Covid-19, the tree was now a problem, and the antidote arrived in the form of a lorry-load of tree surgeons, who reduced it to a large stump. Happily, the tree stump is now sprouting green shoots and promises to form, in due course, a new dome. It will be a long time before a falling branch could cause any damage, but the possibility should not be forgotten.

Although technically we have been partially released from the 'bubble', they continue to figure literally and as a shower of real bubbles – perhaps blown by a child – floats past my window, I can only admire their beautiful rainbow colours and feel light-hearted at their carefree progress. Queen Alexandra is still here and her interests continue to engross me, among them her liking for watching goldfish in their tank. Perhaps we, too, should be inspired by the goldfish, which follows all the rules. It is isolated, but communicates, takes exercise and washes everything, constantly. It can see out and there is fresh air coming in at the top. True, there is the possible danger from the long furry arm of a passing cat, but this may never happen. We hope it does not.

> Merrily blowing bubbles,
> A-swim within the bowl –
> The goldfish plays a leading
> And unexpected role.

CAROL ANN DUFFY

Chosen by Susie Coreth as a poem with particular poignancy, ten years after it was written.

– Silver Lining –
2010

Five miles up the hush and shoosh of ash,
   yet the sky is as clean as a white slate –
I could write my childhood there. Selfish
to sit in this garden listening to the past –
a Tudor bee wooing its flower, a lawnmower –
when the grounded planes mean ruined
      plans, holidays
on hold, sore absences from weddings, funerals,
wingless commerce.
                        But Britain's birds
sing in this spring, from Inverness to Liverpool,
from Crieff, Caernarfon, Cambridge,
      Wenlock Edge,
Land's End to John O' Groats; the music
      silence summons,
George Herbert heard, Burns, Edward Thomas;
      briefly, us.

– Your adventure | A reply to
'An Adventure' by Louise Glück –

A pigeon shat on my hair in the afternoon whilst
I was gardening
So clearly they are lying when people say it brings
good luck
Because your call came a few hours later, long
after sunset

Driving through the night to the hospital
The street lights carried us down the motorway
A battalion of forerunners leading the way to
your bedside

As usual my brain complained with pain
Each pump of blood brings a fresh throb above my
left eye
Whilst each beat of your ventricles forced yet
more of your life through the tear in your aorta

Heart to heart we were locked in a race to see you,
But no one knows how long it will take for you to
bleed out

You've been ill for so long and missed so much
The kaleidoscopic dance floor of birthday parties,
   my graduation and wedding
And now you'll never meet any of your great
   nieces or nephews
When they come to take their place in this world

It occurs to me that you might meet them on the
   other side
Amongst the stars and the rest of the dead,
Once their average of 81.2 years have passed
   on earth.

But you believe that there is only everlasting
   nothingness after death
This world, now pickled in morphine, is all there
   is to you

So I'll keep watch at your bedside and pray you
   find a place amongst the stars
I can feel the dead cheering you on, it's time to
   meet them

Aren't you excited to see your mother again?
No, you don't believe you will

The room fills with the smell of human death
It's new to me and it turns my stomach with
    every inhale
A sweet, rotten cherry rolling from your mouth
With every word, sigh or laboured breath

Now I can taste death everywhere
And catch whiffs of his smell with the slightest
    turn of my head
Even my spliff tastes of you
Stroking the back of my throat during the inhale
    I'm using to temporarily forget you.
But instead you're touching my tonsils

Then I shake myself to
Remembering everything that must be done
And call my dad to get the details of the undertaker,
Ready to take you to the ground when you should
    be amongst the stars.

– Curve Ball –

August 2021

Talk about a curve ball. As humans, we have a natural desire to have control of our lives. Lack of control is scary, unknown and – 2020's word of the year – unprecedented. The pandemic took this from us all in many ways. We live in an age of convenience and suddenly we were stockpiling loo roll and unable to get key ingredients we'd previously taken for granted. Life is full of curve balls, but this one was one that affected everyone across the globe.

I, like most others, was pretty anxious in the early days. I was deemed 'vulnerable' as a paraplegic and suddenly, for the first time in many years, I felt that my disability did indeed leave me exposed and vulnerable to this virus. Having spent the ten years since breaking my back striving to not let my spinal cord injury (SCI) define me, to break down barriers and defy expectations, I realised that I needed to take precautions and protect myself. Chest infections can be fatal for someone with a higher level of injury; therefore this coronavirus did not sound like something I wanted to risk getting.

Feeling extremely fortunate to continue working

from home, I got into the swing of things, and was boosted by my role in the mentoring team at the charity for which I work – connecting people who wanted support from others who had been in a similar situation. Lockdown had a huge effect on people with newly sustained spinal cord injuries, with many not receiving full rehab, not being able to see their families for extended periods and, after discharge, not being able to access the usual opportunities I was fortunate enough to experience, which are absolutely essential in enabling people to see that life is far from over post injury. Consequently, I felt a sense of purpose, which kept my spirits up.

In many ways, lockdown was a leveller for people. At the beginning, we were all worried about loo roll and groceries, the wealthy couldn't jet off on a beach escape and one walk a day was eventually what we were permitted. People were exploring alternative ways to fill their time. Sewing was my activity for a time, my cousin pressed beautiful flowers and sales of childhood favourite, UNO, had unexpectedly surged.

Having said this, it goes without saying that the pandemic exposed, and in some cases heightened, existing inequalities in society. The effects of the pandemic hit those unable to work from home, putting their jobs at risk and reducing their income. Devastatingly, Covid had a greater impact on people with disabilities and people from minority ethnic groups in terms of mortality as well.

For me, it was time to produce the podcast I'd been preparing to put out on to the airwaves. In the month before the pandemic, I'd recorded the first two episodes and then Covid struck, but the silver lining emerged for me in that recording it remotely, and editing it myself, was much more convenient and meant that I could record with anyone, all over the world, regardless of location.

Each week I interviewed an individual who had been through some challenge or adversity in their lives, with the view of helping listeners who were facing their own challenges. At the end of each episode I would ask them for a piece of advice. It is this advice, from these nineteen individuals so far, that has fundamentally changed my attitude and outlook on the world.

It was an absolute privilege to have conversations with such impressive people, from Baroness Tanni Grey-Thompson, TV stars Charley Boorman and George Robinson and Shadow Minister for Women and Equalities MP Marsha de Cordova.

A common theme that emerged for me is actually how well many of the people I knew, who'd been through a life-changing experience like mine, were coping. We'd been through extended periods of isolation, many of us have been forced to sit with and get to know ourselves, and if sustaining my spinal cord injury taught me one thing, it was how to be truly resilient.

The timing of my first series was ideal for me. I was able to have some of the most moving conversations of my life, and to put them out into the world for others to benefit from. I learned about taking responsibility from Paralympic champions; I learned about getting to know yourself from Netflix's *Sex Education* star, George Robinson – a powerful thing at a time when that is all you have, besides your piled up loo roll once you'd acquired your stash; and I learned about reframing and finding gratitude in the darkest of places.

Inspirational podcasts, crafts and UNO aside, the impact of the pandemic has affected the world in far more ways than we could ever have imagined. One of those ways is our mental health. According to the charity, Mind, two-thirds (65 per cent) of adults and three-quarters (75 per cent) of young people with experience of mental health problems said their mental health has become worse during lockdown. Over half of adults (51 per cent) and young people (55 per cent) without experience of mental health problems also said their mental health has got worse during this period.

We know that mental health does not discriminate. The effects of the pandemic are being felt long after we are no longer 'locked down' – people are talking about it, which can only be a positive, but the mental health 'epidemic' is very real. I've certainly witnessed it through my work in speaking to service users, the demand for mentoring increased over lockdown and the waiting list has never been longer during my three-and-a-half years with the team at the charity, Back Up.

Over the course of lockdown, I personally had a rollercoaster of a year, breaking up with my fiancé, buying my first flat and eventually getting a promotion at work. The podcast provided a therapy for me, of sorts, and I was able to seek out guests of my choosing. Thankfully, 10,000+ listeners enjoyed my choices, too.

My conversation with Brett Moran, former crack cocaine addict and convict, now yogi and meditation instructor, was instrumental in setting me on a new path of regularly meditating.

And I enjoyed my conversation with Millie Gooch, founder of Sober Girl Society (a phenomenally successful Instagram account) and author of the Sober Girl Society Handbook, having had the realisation that alcohol was not serving me or giving me what I needed in my life.

So what did I learn? I learned that often when we are going through pain of some sort, it's teaching us something or enabling us to grow, as crappy as it may seem at the time. I learned that it's not anyone else's responsibility to make us happy. It's down to us. We are born alone and we die alone – it's down to us to make shit happen!

Having become paralysed, sustaining a spinal cord injury in 2011 after falling from a roof terrace, something that one often acquires is a level of resilience – breaking my back was the biggest curve ball of all, but if I was going to enjoy my life and get the most out of the hand I'd been dealt, I had to find the strategies to help me do just that.

I learned that resilience can be cultivated by stepping out your comfort zone and embracing failure. I now look for opportunities to step out of this comfort zone, as I know if I'm too comfortable, I'm not growing and learning. And isn't that what life is all about?

Since my SCI, I've become a firm advocate of finding gratitude and having a growth mindset, but during the harder times over the last couple of years I've needed to actively remind myself of this at times (my journal is full of random stuff I'm grateful for – my cat, my comfy bed, voice notes with my best mate), so my advice is to watch out for the good stuff – the blossom on the tree, the good book you're reading, that parking space that's available. For me this year has been a lot about reframing and viewing the situation through a particular lens, in order to serve you best.

After my break up I knew things were going to be hard and so, almost subconsciously, I set about actively managing my mental health. I would religiously go on a walk (push) in my lunchbreak while working from home, 9.00 pm was when my phone went away and it was my new bedtime (or thereabouts, having always been a night owl this took some strength). I binned those bad habits like drinking and smoking, and took actions to keep myself happy.

That's not to say that these 'hacks' can combat clinical depression at all, but certainly in my experience, if you are able, take responsibility as much as you can to give yourself a chance at happiness. It takes effort but, for me, kept me going during what could have been a very dark time.

It has been one of the most challenging times for many of us, but also a time of learning and growth. Life can go at 100mph but lockdown was a chance to slow down and, for many, that was what was needed in order to gain perspective on the important things and what matters most. My guest, Mo Gawdat, talks about the negative bias our brains love to return to time and time again. Even when things seem out of our control, we do have control of where (or with whom) we spend our energy, about where we direct our thoughts, and how we spend our time. This is your responsibility; don't let others dictate those choices, whatever the curve ball you're given might be.

– June 2021 –

I am not convinced that we are quite ready to learn the lessons of lockdown, since it does not seem to be convincingly over. It can never be over until the Government recognises that, henceforth, we must learn to live with Covid as a disease our society has to deal with, and the official bodies still seem a long way off from that.

However, we have learned some lessons certainly since that day, in March 2020, when the lights went out. I was in New York, in pre-production for a series we were about to start shooting, when someone ran into my office (it was about teatime) and told me I would be on the dawn flight back to London, and everything would be suspended. And so I was, and it was. I returned to England the following day, where I was driven down to Dorset, which was where I would play it out. In fact, I probably brought the disease home with me, as a friend rang from America with whom I had recently dined, to say she had been diagnosed, and, at any rate, we all went down with it, which we later had confirmed by our doctor. That was last April, and since now both Emma and I have had our double vaccination shots, I feel as Covid-proof as we can hope to be, and that is rather a comfort.

I don't want to be ambivalent about the period we have just lived through. It has been absolutely terrible for millions of people all around the world. Most obviously for those families who have lost well-loved members, including my own, but also for the many lost livelihoods and shattered educations and economies holed below the waterline, which may recover in the larger sense but which will leave a trail of broken businesses and wasted lives in their wake. In my own business, it is hard to see how some theatres in the provinces will recover, and while some individuals may save themselves by changing horses – I hope they do – it seems that a very central and vibrant part of our cultural history is being undermined and tested to a savage degree.

As a matter of fact, I was a good deal luckier than many in my business, as the series did resume production eventually, and despite the restrictions of Covid filming and travel, necessitating a more elaborate etiquette than Versailles at its height, we got it done. I made two more trips to America, with Covid restrictions, including eating out of boxes on the aeroplane, and so on, but thanks to a tremendous production team and a wonderful cast, it was completed. Added to which, the second *Downton Abbey* film started to shoot a few weeks ago, so I was kept busy. However, life changed, all the same. As it did for everyone. Perhaps as much as anything, in our sense of priorities, and not all the changes were bad. It was not long before that badge of 'Urgent' was dropped from a lot of what I had been planning to do. Clearly, we all had far less in our lives that merited a sense of urgency than we had previously thought. And I regard that as rather liberating.

I enjoyed the sense of a shared crisis that bound the community together. It is not original to compare it with the war, but I remember my mother telling me how, during the war, it felt normal to speak to strangers because you shared a common cause. And although we live in a time when many people seem anxious to dislike anyone who disagrees with them, lockdown was a counter influence to that. For me, we all seemed to feel a need to order from our local pub, to buy in local shops, anything to help them stay afloat.

Of course, I was one of the fortunate ones, of which I am well aware. I chose to spend lockdown at our house in Dorset, which had plenty of room, inside and out, allowing us to live our lives with space and air around us. I say that because my thoughts were often with those in high-rises, possibly with young families needing entertainment, and I thank the Lord that I was not so tested. As a matter of fact, I had a general sense of gratitude that grew out of lockdown. I saw my life from a few steps back, in a way I had not done for a while – if ever – and it was clear to me, to quote Anthony Trollope, my favourite Victorian novelist, that my 'lines had fallen in pleasant places'. I found that I was married to a charming, intelligent and, above all, kind woman, and that my son, the little boy who had so mysteriously been replaced by a thirty-year-old man, had matured into a creative and interesting fellow. I spent more time with them both than I had for ages, and more time with Peregrine than I had since he went away to school in 1999. The truth was our lives had been very full, very busy and very social, with the demands of socialising taking what time was left from work, with house parties and dinner parties and lunches, all boxing and coxing with work duties and filming deadlines. And, while I do not at all mean to complain about any of this, it was oddly welcome to have a time at home, eating together every night, talking about the news, gossiping about the family.

I suppose I have tried to use this episode to think about what it is that I would like to do with the rest of my life. There is a part of me that just wants to get back into the old routine, and I look forward to hearing how bits of my pre-Covid schedule have survived – when will voting go back to normal in the House of Lords, and so on – but there is another voice in my head that tells me this is a unique opportunity, and simply to drift into retirement and old age without thinking it through would be a mistake. What is the work I would still like to have a chance of? Where are the places I would still like to visit? Is there something left to see, to witness, to eat, generally to enjoy? I suppose that is what I would like to take from the whole pandemic year, a sense of something positive that came out of it. That we might have missed if we had just gone on hurtling along in the shuttle car of our life. It does not mean I do not appreciate what people have gone through, but just as my parents brought positive lessons out of a terrible war, if only a desire for positive change, so I would like us to do the same here.

I did not complain before the whole thing came about. As a matter of fact, I believe I have been a lucky person, and I have lived a lucky life. And while it is dangerous and tempting fate to write such things, I feel I have lived the biblical span of three score years and ten. I am seventy-one now, approaching seventy-two, and whatever comes at this point could not re-write the years that have already passed. I've had hit shows and best-selling novels, the thrill of the Oscar stage, the joy of a smash on a Broadway opening night, popular television shows and stage musicals, and generally all the fun of the fair. Lockdown has let me see that, more clearly than I did, and it has perhaps allowed me to feel more blessed. For it is luck and timing, as much as ability, that decides these things, for any number of reasons. So while my heart is with those who have lost loved ones during this time – and my own wife's beloved mother died – despite all this suffering, for myself I find it has also been a time of learning and positive assessment, and that makes me very grateful.

TOM FELTON

– Stuck–

For an outdoor chap, with an outdoor dog
It's never been tricky to find
A reason to run in the sun or the fog
Anything but stuck inside

But alas came the year where it was made clear
That no one should really be out
So we locked the doors, stayed on all fours
And natured the art of the slouch

Moodily did we mooch, just a boy and his pooch
With never any spring in our coil
Ran out of bouncing a ball off the wall
Ran out of frolic and froil

But then came the day, we were freed from
    the cage
And we said goodbye to the roof
Loving life more than ever was everyone, everywhere
Wearing wide smiles as their proof

We celebrated any weather even music
  sounded better
Nothing in life was a chore
Nothing seemed taxing, everyone's relaxing
Long gone the days being bored

More than just surviving, everybody's thriving
Not to be stuck behind door
I'm grateful, so bloody grateful
My dog and I are not stuck inside anymore

– What Have We Done to Ourselves? –
July 2021

In early July 2021, the nature writer Richard Mabey was interviewed on Radio 4. In the course of the year he'd celebrated his eightieth birthday. His writing on nature, and in particular his book, *Nature Cure*, published in 2005, recounts how the natural world can be not just a source of joy and delight, but also a solace and a source of our healing and health. In the course of the interview he made a comment that was quite stark: 'They say that people have been reconnecting to nature and rediscovering it during lockdown.' He then went on to ask, 'So, what have people been doing before lockdown?'

His comment refers to the reality that the human community has, to a degree, been guilty of turning its back on the natural world. At times nature has been seen as an enemy to subdue or a resource to be exploited. Mabey has been, throughout his long writing career, in the vanguard of advocating a deeper sense of reverence for, and appreciation of, the natural world and our place as subjects within nature when at times we have imagined ourselves to be above nature. In recognising nature's power both to heal and to do harm, we are reminded of our human tendency towards hubris.

And, after hubris comes nemesis. The global impact of the Covid-19 pandemic has been a sober reminder of nature's awesome power.

Until only very recently in human history, disease and crop failure would regularly wipe out populations. The constant search for productive land and human anxiety for enough has led generations to migrate across the planet. In the process of 'taming' and 'subduing' nature, we have eliminated countless species and destroyed the habitats of many wild creatures. In addition, we have wrought untold harm to the environment, which has the potential to be catastrophic for the entire Earth community. Some suggest that as we encroach further into the wild places of our world, we are likely to let loose deadly viruses, like Covid-19, which may have been circulating in nature for a long time.

Thomas Carlyle wrote, 'we war with rude nature'. And, of course, you can see where a comment like that comes from. Epidemics like cholera, bubonic plague, typhoid and famine were not a distant memory for Carlyle, who had been aware of the Irish potato famine of the mid-nineteenth century that led to the death of about a million people. Nature can be an enemy and the Covid-19 pandemic is an example. For all our sophistication, technological achievements and global networks, we are not immune from nature's wrath.

As a minister of the Church of Scotland, I am aware of the extent to which my own faith tradition has colluded in a long period of indifference to, and even disdain for, the natural world. In the book of Genesis, we read of the instruction to Adam and Eve to subdue nature. That is in Genesis chapter 1, but in Genesis chapter 2, there is a wholly different perspective, that human beings were put into the Garden to 'tend and serve'. The paradox is that you have in the first two chapters of the Hebrew Bible two wholly different injunctions. Do we subdue and have dominion or tend and serve? Human history, certainly over the last 1,600 years, has tended to err on the side of the former. However, I believe that we are at the beginning of a great sea change. And I believe that our way into a viable future must involve the recovery of a nature-centred spirituality. This is not pantheism – the worship of nature as god – but a recognition that the Divine nature manifests herself through the created order, an idea we have, at times, lost sight of.

Over the years, I have struggled with the Church's theology. The Hebrew Bible can be read like an agricultural manual. The Book of Deuteronomy speaks about resting the land and not over-cropping it, and about responsible animal husbandry as well as provision for the poor. It recognises that human civilisation depends on successful agriculture. Get your agriculture right and the human community will thrive; get it wrong and civilisation will collapse. In spite of this truth, the Christian church is something of a latecomer to the environmental movement.

In the New Testament, there is a real sense of Jesus having arisen from peasant stock. He alludes constantly to the patterns of the natural world and tells stories and parables about agricultural practices. Indeed, it is on his rare visits to the city that he encounters his keenest opposition. In the great city of Jerusalem, the ecclesiastical and political authorities of the day collude to bring his ministry to an abrupt end. Jesus has been described as a 'rural redeemer' and man of the soil, at home not so much in the corridors of power but grubbing around in the dirt and rhythms of rural Galilee.

When Christianity became the official religion of the Roman Empire in the fourth century, it adopted the clothes of empire, including an urbanism that has at times disdained the natural world. The structure of the Christian church and its theology since the fourth century has been overwhelmed by patterns that are often more associated with the exercise of power than with the ideas of both the Hebrew people as a pastoral community and Jesus, who was deeply rooted in rural culture, aware of the patterns of the natural world.

There is one part of 'Christendom' that evaded this movement: the Celtic peoples. It might even be accurate to say that just as the Romans failed fully to conquer Scotland and Ireland, so the ideas that went with the Christian Empire failed to take root within the Celtic tradition.

At one time the Celtic peoples extended from Turkey to the Atlantic coast. However, as the empire grew – both Roman and later the Christian Empire – the Celtic peoples were pushed further and further west, so that today they inhabit only the Atlantic fringe of Europe. At various times not just the Celtic people's but Celtic Christianity was suppressed and opposed by the Church.

I have always been drawn to what some people describe as Celtic spirituality. However, there are many within my faith community that pour scorn of those of us that take an interest in this tradition. We have been variously accused of heresy and dabbling in dangerous magic and straying from the orthodox belief of the Church. There is, however, a whole movement of scholars, poets, artists and thinkers within the Celtic fringe who keep alive many of the traditions and perspectives that have their roots on the edge of empire, untainted by many of the attitudes that have characterised both the Roman and Christian Empires that have dominated Europe since Constantine the Great embraced Christianity in the fourth century.

Within the Celtic tradition the relationship between faith and nature has been maintained. My own Church of Scotland has often felt like an institution of modernity with a structure that has, at times, been overly preoccupied with perpetuating itself, only having regard for the salvation of individual human souls and not thinking much at all about the natural world. In addition, there have been times in our recent past when the Church of Scotland has colluded in the suppression of not just Celtic culture but also the language and traditions of our Gaelic and Celtic heritage.

Celtic spirituality acts as a counter to those who have viewed nature merely as a resource at the disposal of human beings, to be used, manipulated and discarded, but of no intrinsic worth. As people rediscover nature and, through this time, reflect on nature's power, it feels right to reassess our attitudes to the natural world and to learn a deeper appreciation. The writer and spiritual activist, Alastair McIntosh, said to me recently, 'Celtic spirituality is about reopening blocked wellsprings that give life.' In a world traumatised and shaken by a natural phenomenon like the pandemic, there is a reawakening going on.

So, I ask the question, what have we done to ourselves?

The answer is that for the best part of 1,600 years we have pushed ourselves further and further way from a connection to the natural world. In our building of empires and plundering of the earth we have, at times, forgotten that we are subjects within nature and not masters of it.

Richard Mabey reminds us that connecting with nature can be immensely therapeutic. During lockdown, life paused long enough for many of us to reconnect and to find the natural world a source of healing and joy. The pandemic also revealed to us that nature can be harsh and indifferent to human suffering. She demands of us a respect and reverence that invites us not to work against her but to work with her.

In the Celtic spiritual tradition, that clings on at the very fringe of Europe, I believe there are the seeds of a wisdom about how to recover a more appropriate relationship with nature. Reverence, awe and wonder will lead to a deeper respect for nature. Our lack of respect is what has led to the current climate emergency and this global health emergency reminds us of the need to reimagine our relationship with the natural world on which we depend.

The great physicist, Stephen Hawking, amongst many others in the scientific community said recently that the greatest causes of climate change are greed, indifference and selfishness. Science has a lot to say about how we might technically fix some of the challenges we face, one of which is certainly how we deal with the occurrence of pandemics in the future as we encroach more and more into the world's wild places and become more and more globally connected. However, the one thing that science is powerless to do anything about, he declared, is human greed, indifference and selfishness. These are spiritual challenges. A recovery of a spiritual tradition that more fully takes account of the natural world will surely help, and much of the wisdom needed for that renewal, lies within the ancient Celtic spiritual tradition.

Through this strange time, many people who thought they had outgrown the need for prayer and spirituality have found themselves returning to them, exploring meaning and purpose, and re-visiting nature. Richard Mabey may well ask, 'Where have you been all these years of your heedless life?' I'm sure that people have not lost faith and a deep-rooted search for spiritual meaning; it is just that they have, at times, lost faith in the institutions of religion that can seem over-preoccupied with themselves than with the world.

So, out of the Celtic fringe, squeezed as it has been to the edge, is ancient wisdom to be rediscovered and shared that will help heal the rift that has grown up between humanity and the natural world. Of course, the current pandemic is not nature's judgement on heedless humanity, but it is a reminder that we cannot rise above our natural state.

Our way into the future has to be one that relies on the application of good and responsible science, but also recovers that spiritual dimension to life that sees glory, wonder and awe in the natural world of which we are part. The Celtic fringe has much to teach this generation about restraint, respect and reverence.

I conclude with two wise sayings from the Celtic fringe of Europe.

The first from Pierre Teilhard De Chardin:

The day will come when, after harnessing space, the winds, the tides and gravitation, we shall harness for God the energies of love. And on that day, for the second time in the history of the world, we shall have discovered fire.

The second is a blessing from St Columba:

Be thou a bright flame before me,
Be thou a guiding star above me,
Be thou a smooth path below me,
Be thou a kindly shepherd behind me,
Today, tonight, and for ever more.

– Eight Bottles in an Oak Tree –

It was a Thursday afternoon when I first heard it. I woke up that morning feeling very lazy. I meant to go running at 8.00 am. Before breakfast. Before Mum could delay me. Before I decided I didn't want to anymore. However, 8.00 quickly became 9.00, which all of a sudden was noon and then it was lunchtime. So I waited. It was 2.30 pm or so when I finally left. A relaxed 5km was the goal. Running the loop that leads me through the fields. An open blue sky above me. Nothing to shield me from the sun and it was sweltering. My feet were pounding the road, feeling heavier than normal. I was so slow that day.

STACY.

I heard it calling my name as I rounded that third corner. The one by the apple trees. Somewhere between kilometre 3 and 4.

STACY.

I stopped. Had I imagined it?

STACY.

I couldn't see anyone. I looked up. I don't think it was God. I feel like there would have been some dark and stormy rain clouds or something. Or at least some lightning. I paused. I didn't respond. Didn't want to look like a maniac.

Nothing. I kept running.

Curious, I ran the same loop the next day. I went at the same time.

STACY.

Right as I was passing the apple trees.

STACY. LOOK LEFT.

There was a rather large oak tree. I'm so sure it hadn't been there before. I thought, for a second, I might've seen a pair of eyes staring back out of the hole in the trunk, but I got spooked and kept going.

I tried to avoid the route from then on but, for some reason, I went back today. I don't know why. Actually, I do. She'd been at me again. Mum, I mean. I'd had to move back home because of coronavirus. I love her, but she'd been driving me round the bend. What are you going to do with your life, Stacy? No one is going to hire you with half a degree. Why did you break up with Clara, Stacy? She was such a nice girl. So sweet. How are you going to support yourself now, Stacy? You can't live at home forever.

STACY.

She kept asking. So I got up, put on my shoes and ran. I ran as fast as I could to the tree.

STACY.

I don't know what I want to do with my life. Why did I decide to study maths in the first place? You told me to, that's why. It was what I was good at, I suppose. Because she fucking cheated on me, Mum, in the middle of a pandemic, when we weren't supposed to be seeing anyone anyway and how did she manage to do that without me noticing, you might ask and fair enough, this is also a question I've asked myself many times and –

The third question then. I have no idea, not a clue. No money. No girlfriend. No career. Not even my flat to live in anymore. So I went running to the tree because it was calling my name.

STACY. LOOK LEFT.

The tree was on fire. No, really. On. Fire. But I couldn't smell anything. There was no ash, no smoke. Just flames.

YOU'RE READY NOW.

The eyes appeared in the trunk of the tree again. They were bright purple – very obvious amongst the yellow flames that were making their way down the trunk. I made my way over, jumping over the ditch that ran along the side of the road, picking through the brambles that seemed immune to the flames. I could just about make out a face. Was it a squirrel?

TOUCH THE FIRE.

I'd come this far, hadn't I? I reached out and touched the flames. And felt nothing. They weren't hot. They weren't cold. They weren't ... anything really. It didn't feel any different. I reached further. I suddenly felt a pull behind my belly button, like someone had hooked me on to a very large fishing rod and was pulling me upwards. My feet left the ground which had now started to spin. I was tumbling through space. I could make out objects around me, but they weren't clear enough to identify. I became very aware that I couldn't move. Before I could think too much more about this, my butt hit the ground and I was now sitting with my back against something hard. Wood.

STACY.

I looked up to see a small figure emerging from the shadows. It was a small boy.

'Hugo?'

Hugo had been my neighbour. His parents had moved about a year after his death. We were both five or six at the time. We'd just started school. He'd been on a swing set in the garden when the chain had snapped. I remember my mum explaining what a coma was to me at the time. I didn't understand how the sleep could be bad for him. I'd loved sleep. Why was it bad? Why couldn't they just let him sleep? But sometimes people never wake up, my mum had explained. Her voice soft as she said it. She had been stroking my hair. He died two weeks later.

YES.

'What on earth are you doing here?'

WELL, IT IS ME. AND IT'S NOT ME. HUGO
IS WHAT YOU SEE. SO HUGO I AM.

I haven't thought about Hugo in years.

WHAT DO YOU NEED, STACY?

'Ummm. What?'

WHAT DO YOU NEED?

I shook my head.
    'You called me here. Why am I here? I want to
ask the questions.'

ONLY THOSE WHO NEED THE OAK SEE
THE OAK.

'Right. This is a magic tree.'

NO, MAGIC DOESN'T EXIST.

'Okay. What would you call this?'

DESPERATION.

The little boy smiled as he said this last word.

'Hey now –'

YOU SAW THE TREE WHEN YOU
NEEDED THE TREE.

So I created a magic tree powered by desperation. Excellent. If that didn't just sum up 2020.

WHAT DO YOU NEED?

Hugo asked again. Now that I thought about it, I was fairly thirsty. I'd sprinted those 3km to the tree. Nothing quite like rage to get you to run fast.

'Water, I suppose?'

Eight bottles of water appeared in front of me. The tall glass bottles resembled the kind you would get in a fancy restaurant trying to be hipster. Each one was a different bright colour.

'Is that safe to drink?'

DEPENDS ON YOUR DEFINITION OF SAFE.

'Will I die?'

EVENTUALLY, YES.

I rolled my eyes. This little version of Hugo was

sassy. Though, he had been that way before. Even at six, he was funny, quick thinking. He was the one who had wanted to switch out his brother's birthday cake for mud, and he'd made the whole thing work. It had been brilliant.

'What are these?'

THEY WILL EACH GIVE YOU WHAT YOU NEED.

'What does that mean?'

I was still leaning against the wood. I hadn't moved at all. My hands were hanging limp by my side. As I thought about them, my fingers seemed to remember that they existed. I wiggled one. It wiggled back. I lifted them up to examine them. They looked okay. I used one of my newly discovered hands and reached out for the first bottle. I uncorked it.

ARE YOU REALLY GOING TO SWIG STRAIGHT FROM THE BOTTLE?

'I don't have a glass.'

One appeared.

'Yeah, because that's not magic.'

YOU NEEDED ONE.

'Alright. Can I just taste it?'

YOU MUST CHOOSE.

'But how do I know what I'm choosing?'

PAY ATTENTION, STACY.

Well that rankled a bit. Mum was always saying that to me. When I walked into furniture or knocked over the wine bottle on the table. When I'd almost forgotten to reply to a job offer. That had been bad. When I'd stayed in bed for three days. She'd sat down at the foot of the bed and looked at me.

'Your whole life is happening in front of you, love,' Mum had said. 'Pay better attention.'

I picked up the bottle. It was a very subtle shade of pink. As I looked closer, the water started to swirl, creating colours and shapes. I could see ... wait, was that Clara? There she was. Standing in the living room of our flat. I could see her putting up Christmas decorations. She looked so happy. This was ridiculous. Christmas was months away. And we'd long ago both moved out. And then – that was me! I walked into the picture and her arm was around me.

IF YOU DRINK THAT, CLARA WILL NEVER HAVE CHEATED.

Hugo's voice made me jump. I wanted to be in that living room. I wanted to be putting up Christmas decorations. I wanted –

Hang on.

'But does that mean she didn't want to? Or she wouldn't?'

IT CAN'T PREDICT THE FUTURE.

'But I'll know she might. I can't –'

She'd told me while I was brushing my teeth. Some girl who'd followed her on Instagram. I had just kept brushing my teeth, not sure what to do. Her voice had come in one ear and my brain had taken that information and buried it deep inside of me. I could feel it now.

'No!'

But it was too late. I was crying. I couldn't stop. I threw the bottle into the darkness.

I TAKE IT YOU DON'T WANT THAT ONE THEN.

The bottle didn't make a sound. It just disappeared

into the shadows. I had wanted it to crash. I had wanted it to break. Hugo stared at me while my sobbing slowed.

TRY ANOTHER ONE.

The second bottle was tinted green. I could see my mum. We were seated side by side on my bed. She was holding my hand.

'I suppose my mum and I are best friends in this one then.'

For some reason, that seemed a bit simple to me.

YES.

Did I want that? I wasn't sure.

DO YOU NEED IT?

I looked at him. I wasn't sure of that either. I put it back.

The bright yellow bottle had numbers floating around in the water.

MATHS.

'That means I go back to my degree?'

As I said the words, I knew it wasn't that bottle that I wanted. Or needed. I didn't even want to pick it up.

TRY BOTTLE NUMBER FIVE.

'I didn't know you had opinions.'

But I picked it up. I was sitting on a swing. As I stared into this one (a shade of aquamarine) I could see a boy walk up to me. He was tall. Vaguely familiar. He held out something in his hand. It looked like a brownie. The me on the swing looked very suspicious and then started to laugh. She took it and crumbled it in her hand. Mud.

'Hugo?'

YES.

'In this one, you're not dead.'

YES.

'I can't do that. Can I? Wouldn't that upset the balance of the Force or something? Even if it's not magic, someone can't just come back to life, can they?'

The bottle started to grow warm in my hand. The water started to bubble.

'Hugo, what's going on?'

YOU DON'T BELIEVE.

The bottle was scorching me now but I couldn't seem to let go.

'Hugo – help me!'

He backed away into the shadows.

BELIEVE.

'I AM SITTING AT THE BOTTOM OF A TREE THAT IS ON FIRE TALKING TO A DEAD SIX-YEAR-OLD, I DEFINITELY FUCKING BELIEVE!'

I took a breath. It was so hot. I was starting to sweat. I could still make out the grown-up Hugo sitting down on the swing next to me.

HURRY.

I didn't know what to do. It was really starting to hurt. My fingers were glued to the bottle. I closed my eyes and I tried to throw it. It didn't budge. I tried again. On the third go, I felt the bottle leave my hand and fly into the shadows. Blisters had formed on the palm of my hand that had been holding on to the bottle.

YOU CAN'T BRING BACK THE DEAD.

'But then why –'

HE MIGHT BE WHAT YOU NEED.

'But then why – I know I can't – I don't –'

I hadn't thought about Hugo in so long. I missed him. Afterwards. And no one asked. No one asked me about him. So I'd forced myself to forget. Those memories of him played across my mind, quick flashes of childhood memories.

THAT'S HUGO'S STORY, THOUGH.

'So do I need him?'

THAT'S NOT A CHOICE YOU GET TO MAKE.

The bottle was gone. Its space stood empty, and I couldn't see beyond the shadows behind the small figure.

I reached for another bottle; it was a tame cream colour. Mum would probably call it something stupid like 'off-cream-broken-egg-shell'. I was running. That's all I could see as I held it up to my face. Inside the bottle, I was running.

'Explain this one to me.'

YOU ARE RUNNING.

'Yes, I see that.'

YOU CAN RUN FAST.

'Is that all?'

VERY FAST.

Before my brain quite realised what I was doing, I uncorked the bottle, reached for the glass, and poured the water and drank. It tasted like water. Nothing special about it. I poured a second glass and drank that quickly too. I really had been very thirsty. I looked over at Hugo.

WELL DONE.

He started to fade. I couldn't quite make out the edges of him anymore.

'Hugo?'

Silence. The world started to spin again. I could feel that space behind my belly button yank upwards. And then I was standing on the road again. Looking at an empty space where the oak had been.

How in the –

I looked out at the road ahead. And I started to run. And wow. I could really run. Faster than I had ever run. It wasn't easier, necessarily, but something tangible had changed. As I ran, I thought about Hugo. I thought about the real Hugo. I hadn't in so long. I thought about sitting on those swings and unpacking the world in all the ways we knew how at six years old. I thought about Clara and what she had done to me. I thought about brushing my teeth that day. Not being able to cry immediately, because my mouth had been full of toothpaste. I thought about my mum and those questions she had asked. I thought about the answers to them. Or the fact that I didn't have answers to them. I could feel them as I ran, all of those thoughts in my head. I ran and the thoughts slowed down. So, I kept on running.

– June 2021 –

Over lockdown I began running through central London in the evenings. I'm not fit but I can run slowly in a straight line – and the centre of town was stunning and empty. I began running past my favourite places – only working out what they were as I went. Most nights I slowed down to pay my respects to the London Library, a gentler deeper internet, where you could, in normal times, borrow books that hadn't been touched since 1955. I ran through Chinatown; the lights were on but nobody was there. Westminster Abbey stood as lonely as a country church. London will never feel the same again.

Throughout this period, we have missed birthdays. Or rather they have passed unconfirmed and acknowledged. As have bereavements. My father died abroad, in the midst of lockdown, so I attended his funeral on Zoom. The mourners took their places in rows on the screen. One of my father's oldest friends joined the Zoom call from a restaurant in America – and just as the coffin was being lowered into the ground, she pressed a button on her phone and took over the screen.

The rest of us watched transfixed as she slowly and loudly ordered a margarita.

Back in February 2020, I knew how to manage in the world. I could negotiate the bus, the shops and most other people. Not now. I'm taking very few tasks for granted these days. Last week, in a public building, I walked into the men's toilets. The urinals were out of action for social distancing reasons, cordoned off with black-and-yellow police tape. I stepped, instead, into a cubicle and found its door missing. Ah, right, I thought, this must be a Covid rule. No more toilet doors. Another new thing. After four or five seconds I pulled myself together. Every other cubicle had its door. Mine just happened to be missing. We *weren't* now supposed to defecate publicly in front of each other like wartime soldiers in a makeshift camp. However, I had been willing to believe – *for an appreciable length of time* – that we were.

Ten years from now, I'll want to relive some Covid memories more than others. Above all, I hope, I'll remember my evening runs through the city. They were bursts of freedom borne out of restriction. They were wonderfully enjoyable and entirely unexpected. Forget the rules, the queues, the masks, the road rage, Zoom and the virus itself. Never again will the world – or London, at least – be left to darkness and to me.

– The Heart's Engagements –

I.

For every lover who might be convinced
His happiness was always meant to be,
A discovery awaits; the heart's engagements,
For all their script of perfect sunsets
Are arbitrary and unplanned, except
In the most grimly fatalistic
Of philosophies – those systems
That leave us not much of a say
In what becomes of us, or of others.
Love is an accident, and like
Just about every accident, it occurs
When you are doing something else,
Collecting the shopping, walking to work,
Or innocently reading the newspaper.
Love is never timely; love never arrives
According to the timetable, like an Italian
Railway train under autocratic government.

II.

Nor is love a matter of desert:
The undeserving and the selfish
May be loved by the kind and considerate;
Those of unmerchantable quality,
By any standards, may still attract
The attention of the discerning
And the gifted; bad matches
May turn out well after all,
As when the bully or the brute
Discovers kindness and a perfect angel
Who softens a hardened heart,
And makes of him a kindly lover:
That happens, sometimes, in books.

III.

Love has never been a matter of fairness,
Aphrodite's reputation, such as it is,
Was never based on having an eye
For what is right and choosing accordingly:
Her young and naked bowman
Has an aim that can be haphazard,
Even if his misplaced darts
Are occasionally welcome where they land;
Love is governed by roulette-odds:

Depends on a profile, or a look,
Having nothing to do, in so many cases,
With temperament or ability
To empathise – that is everything to do
With friendship, which is a field
Into which Eros is not meant to wander.
Friendship ripens into love but is not
The sort of love that makes us ache,
Behave unreasonably, or mope
Around the house for days on end;
Friendship makes us do none of that.

IV.

What we hope for in love, at least
When we have had enough experience
To know the way that it works,
Is acceptance – of our faults
Our limitations, our failure to be
All that others would like us to be;
Love understands, rather than judges,
Reassures the least of us; convinces us
That we are not alone; allows the use
Of the first-person plural
When the single form is just too lonely:
We and *us* have always been more natural
To a social species than *I* and *me*.

V.

Finding love is never easy,
Except for those who, blessed
With beauty, make it seem
Effortless and expected;
We all know one who has only to smile
And hearts are broken;
Oddly, love eludes some like them,
Love's tributes lie at their feet,
But may seem empty, undeserved;
Garlands wilting and ignored
Because they fell too easily, perhaps.

VI.

Girls may fall in love with one another,
And the same is true of boys,
Love is indifferent to the conventions
Of chromosomes; Jonathan and his David
Were touching in their devotion,
In their hills and high places,
And today, after long years
Of disapproval and unkindness
We see that it hardly matters:
Boy meets boy and girl meets girl
Is nothing to be embarrassed about:

All love is the same delight
In another; keeping a name
Upon lips gives us pleasure
Whatever that name may be.

VII.

Of all the themes by which
A writer lives, love unrequited
Is one of the greatest, there is
Something noble about those
Who nurture a passion for another
Who cannot or who will not
Reciprocate their love:
One of the great subjects of literature
Is nevertheless, for those involved,
A sad business of tissues
Soaked with tears, of bleakness,
Of long waiting for a sign that never comes:
Pity the unrequited love that never is.

VIII.

We may lose the one we love
In so many and such different ways,
All of them, it seems to us,
At the time of loss at least,

Uniquely, personally cruel, and undeserved;
Affection may wane, just as we go off
A cardigan we used to like
Or a painting we've grown out of;
Another may catch our lover's eye
With offers we can never match –
Novelty, for one; or oceans
May intervene between us:
It is hard for one in San Francisco
To love another in Mozambique
Even with electronic assistance;
Or the one we love may simply go away;
That happens too, and may be irreversible.
And yet love shares with Persephone,
With Diana, and all the rest,
A certain immortality; love persists
In memory, and is always there,
Ready to remind us of what it was we had,
A quiet, insistent whisper in the heart.

LEON McCARRON

– Three Miles an Hour –
August 2021

In January 2020 I drove for three hours from Erbil to Sulaymaniyah across the Kurdistan region of Iraq. It rained heavily, fat drops on the window smudging the road into grey sky, and the next day the temperature dropped enough for precipitation to turn to snow. I left my car in lieu of walking boots and a heavy jacket, and with a small group of shivering friends made for the mountains. Thick-set canyons were softened by falling flakes, and a deafening wind hid from us the roar of a waterfall until we were almost upon it. We clambered along narrow trails, over rock washed clean by the storm, and farther still until we found the recess of a long, wide cave. Our joy at the respite was proportional to the peace and silence of that place, and we stayed a long time, watching mountains come and go behind a wall of weather.

Walking has been my companion for much of the last decade, and I have travelled perhaps 10,000 miles on foot in that time. If that sounds like a lot, it hasn't felt it, because each step was so simple, so effortless. I have set out again and again, waiting to fall into a cadence, and it is the only way I know to align body and mind together so that they move as one. That, in turn, opens the doors for everything else to happen along the way.

Walking has many functions, and I've come to think of it primarily as a catalyst for understanding. It reveals much that otherwise gets lost by the unnatural speed at which we so often move and, above all, it can show how one place, one conversation, one idea, is connected to the next. On a long walk each new experience is bonded to the last and fused to what follows. Realising this has helped me reimagine the planet we live on.

Since 2017 I have been designing a long-distance walking trail across the Kurdish region in northern Iraq. This involves finding, researching and walking the old ways of the land, and joining them together to reimagine their function as part of a journey. Trails bring people together, placing strangers side by side, and encourage an exchange between those who inhabit and those who visit. The structure removes many of the risks that some might associate with walking, or in this case with walking Iraq, and makes the experience of discovery at three miles an hour accessible to many. Kurdistan, a semi-autonomous region in the north of Iraq with a population of 7 million, may seem an unlikely place for these ambitions, given the recent history of the country. It should not be, and my hope is that in the future it will be seen for what it is and can be, rather than what it was, or what people fear it to be. To me it is a vast furrowed landscape, latticed with paths and layered with history, culture and faith. Occasional villages sparsely populate the wilderness and hidden in the wrinkles are coiled gorges and alpine meadows. On my first visit to Kurdistan, I was fortunate to meet a young man called Laween Mohammed who bounced rather than walked. He is a prodigious hiker who steps always with a smile and Laween and I have walked perhaps 800 miles together, stitching together ancient footpaths through the Zagros Mountains.

Kurdistan became my permanent home in 2019, but when the pandemic hit, I got stuck in the UK. Borders closed and it became clear there would be no return for quite some time. I don't suppose any of us spent the last year the way we had planned; all I really know is that I was one of the lucky ones. Surrounded by loved ones, I was healthy and I could still walk, albeit restricted to the same track of a few miles. I was reminded of the great guru of stillness, Pico Iyer, who said that 90 per cent of his life was spent at a desk writing about the 10 per cent when he was more active. To even consider travel felt improper for so long, but when my mind did wander it was not to new places; it was to those mountains that I'd left behind.

It was autumn 2020 before I returned. Businesses had re-opened and travel into the region was restarting. I flew back to Erbil to live and to assess the impact of the pandemic on the more remote sections of trail. Laween and I would check in on our colleagues, help where possible and strategise for the future.

While it was remarkable to be moving again, we had to be certain we would not be risking transmission of the virus to those we met. Our team was tested every two days, and we wore masks and socially distanced. Our local colleagues did the same, and we did not stay in homes as we used to. The responsibilities and privileges of travellers have finally come into sharper focus in the last year, and the pandemic accentuates the questions that we all must ask ourselves when we move: Why are we here? What are we trying to achieve? Who is really benefiting?

The old town of Akre is built into the fold at the foot of a mountain and above the central bazaar houses climb haphazardly upwards, finally running out of steam halfway to the top. On a clear

November day, Laween and I met with a shepherd called Sadiq Zebari, whose perpetual frown belies a sweet disposition. Sadiq has spent weeks guiding us here and told us that almost everyone he knew had caught Covid-19. It had been tough, and now he wanted to walk. There's a certain unspooling that follows the slowness and considered nature of climbing a hill, and conversations with Sadiq only really began after a few miles at such a pace.

Together we wheezed up to the ridgeline about the town, leaning on one another at the corners of the switchback, and at the top Sadiq lay out flat and stared up to space, smoking cigarette after cigarette. His own experience of the virus was brief but brutal. 'The fever was so bad,' he said, 'that every night I rode my motorcycle to a spring at midnight and jumped in fully clothed.' The spring was known locally to cure illnesses, and he was sure that this is why it only took him one week to recover. He went under the cover of darkness because during the lockdown the police had restricted all non-essential movement outside of homes. Above all, Sadiq has missed the freedom to roam whenever he wanted. 'Freedom and cigarettes,' he sighed, 'that's all I ever need.'

Northeast, in the lush Barzan valley, our friend Anwar Safti said that most of his village of 200 families got sick. 'I had pain from my head to my feet,' he said. 'I didn't walk for two months, and it was like my brain stopped working.' Farther along, where the spine of the vast Bradost Mountain curves inwards and squeezes the Great Zab River into ever-narrower gorges, we walked with our wiry colleague, Jawad Qamaryan, from his village to a high pass. Jawad is a man of the mountains and hopped lightly across the rocks as we heaved our city-heavy legs behind. 'Ah, the virus from China,' he said after some initial confusion. 'No-one here has had it.'

No-one? 'I heard some bad stories from Erbil, but here it didn't bother us.' The schools had closed, we learned, but little else changed. 'Villages like ours are clever,' said Jawad. 'We keep everything local anyway. If I can't go to Erbil, no problem. Who wants to go to the big city anyway?'

It will likely be years before we know why there seem to be so many inconsistencies in how and where this virus spreads. Cities in the Kurdistan region suffered terribly. Laween witnessed that first-hand. However, in the villages, it was more unpredictable. Some saw widespread infection, others barely any at all. In Choman, by the Iranian border, we heard the death rate in hospitals was as high as 10–15 per cent, but just 10 miles to the west, no deaths were reported. There was no discernible difference between the actions of the local population in each place.

What is clear is that, even for Jawad, the virus has altered reality. Maybe one of the few universal truths that we can take from this is that everything has changed. A second could be that existence is fragile. A third, perhaps, is that when we stop moving, the earth beneath us heals. Without doubt the most ubiquitous feedback that we received was how successfully landscape and wildlife had regenerated. 'I've never seen it like this in my lifetime,' said Jawad.

For Anwar Safti, it helps to think about things in terms of a journey on foot. 'This time in the world is like climbing a mountain in winter,' he told us. 'The snow is deep and every step is miserable. We are cold and tired. But we also know that in five, or ten, or twenty hours we will be done. We will be finished, and after that we can go home. Things always change. It's bad, but it will get better. We must trust in that.'

As we all try to regain our footing and work out our next steps, I take solace in those words.

A part of this piece was originally published online by www.adventure.com in March 2021

ANNA MYERS

– Break in the Clouds –

I.

On my boyfriend's bedroom window sill, nestled between the blue ceramic elephant I gave him for his birthday last year and the plant he waters every Sunday without fail, sits a yellow ball of glass I affectionately call his *sunlight spinn-y thing-y*.

The correct name for it would be a Crookes radiometer, and it works like this: inside the glass ball, two tiny silver vanes are mounted on a spindle, which rotates when exposed to sunlight. The more light it receives, the faster it spins. For it to function properly, the vanes need to exist inside a perfect vacuum. In its absence, which is to say if the bulb is full of air, the push of the photons hitting the glass will not be strong enough to move the vanes.

I have long been fascinated by this tiny golden device. No matter how many times I read up on the science behind it, it still feels a bit like magic every time the sun peeks out from under a cloud and the small aluminium squares start spinning faster than my dogs jump when they hear the word *salami*. I have watched the tiny thing slow and then settle down as a storm brews, spin so fast that I thought they'd crash right out of their glass cage on a hot July morning, and sometimes just sit quietly, motionlessly, and wait for a break in the clouds.

I, too, have been waiting for mine.

Lately, like everyone I know and most people I have never met, I have shrunk my life smaller and smaller until it can fit in the space between my bedroom and kitchen. I count in days, sometimes hours. I think in lists. I made a list of books I wanted to read and stacked them all on the first shelf I'd emptied in view of the move, weeks ago when moving house was still an option. That was the last time I touched them. I made a list of all the good things still happening in the world: did you know the canal water in Venice is now so clean that dolphins are swimming in it? I made a list of non-perishable ingredients, brandished it while wandering the aisles of the enormous, empty supermarket two streets down from my house. I didn't buy anything on the list. I rang up a bag of cauliflower florets and three packets of pink fizzy candy instead – I told myself it's because they were on a 3-for-2 discount, but it's really because sugar is comfort, and comfort is all I have right now.

I have a list of movies to watch, webinars to replay,

recipes to cook, friends to call, articles to read and even yoga classes to join on Instagram live. The only thing I stopped listing is how many times I've already checked on my parents, and that's because I start crying every time I think of how long it could still be before I can hug them again. They're locked inside their house in Milan, right at the centre of the Italian red zone, but they're safe and healthy and the dogs are still allowed to sit in the sun on the balcony until the bright light reduces their eyes to tiny slits.

It's the little things, I know.

The thing is, the aluminium vanes exist in a perfect vacuum, but we do not. Individual actions have never mattered more than they do at this moment in time, and we have never been more connected. I jump every time I get a Google News notification after 5.00 pm, because I know that one of them will inevitably contain the daily death stats amongst the latest headlines, and day after day I struggle to make sense of the numbers as they show no sign of slowing down.

I struggle to check in with myself when I know I really should close Twitter after refreshing it for the fourth time in an hour, to check my bank account even though I know there won't be much coming in for a while, and to check on my partner's emotional state after I unload my own barrel of anxieties on him day after day.

However, I check the yellow ball of glass every morning before going down to make coffee. The weather has been uncharacteristically sunny for the past few days, and the squares haven't stopped spinning.

It sits between the blue ceramic elephant and the plant my man waters every Sunday without fail. I tell myself: we will celebrate his birthday again, perhaps at the place around the corner where the carbonara is served in a cheese wheel and tastes exactly like it does back home. Perhaps they'll give us a table by the window, and we'll share the tiramisu. Maybe we'll celebrate it in a different country; the one we were planning to ship all our stuff to in labelled brown boxes, before all this happened.

But we will celebrate it again.

I tell myself: he still waters his plants every Sunday, without fail.

I tell myself: the tiny squares inside the yellow ball of glass start spinning every time the sun peeks out from behind a cloud.

I watch them rotate faster and faster, and I tell myself: comfort is all we have right now.

II.

On Tuesday, on my daily government-allowed walk, I go around the park instead of towards the canal. I take a couple of wrong turns. I walk some more, stop right in front of a church that I'd never noticed before. Partly hidden by foliage, mostly drenched in the atypical April sunshine I've been so grateful for these past few weeks. It stands in the middle of a tiny square, and looking all around it, I don't see anybody else. I haven't seen anybody else in a long time.

I sit on one of the benches and remove my headphones. I'm not sure where God stands on the pop charts these days and I'm not planning to find out. I just stare and stare, up at the rose windows. And look, I'm not religious. Not in any real sense.

But I am not a cynic, either.

And I'm no stranger to the search for something godly.

Early last year, I went through a bad phase. Every single day during my lunch break, I'd sit at the café near my office, claim the corner armchair and order a sandwich with too much cheese and not enough vegetables. I'd feel sick three bites in but would always finish the entire thing. I'd watch *Friends* reruns on my phone for an hour, just so I wouldn't have to *think think think.*

It wasn't the first bad stretch. I've lived through a few. Mostly short-lived ones, with the exception of The Terrible Year That Was 2017, but short-lived is not always synonymous with light. The more powerful ones kicked me in the stomach with such force, such venom, that at times I could barely breathe. I used to live in fear of them, knowing the next one couldn't be too far around the corner.

These days, I am more grateful than scared.

Because it is only thanks to all the bad stretches and all the lunch breaks spent trying not to cry, not to think, not to feel, that I now know how to spot joy when I see it.

My body can't ever forget what it feels like to always be one step removed from your own life; what it feels like when getting out of bed requires more effort than winning the lottery does luck. The bad years were bad for a reason, and I can never get them back, but remembering means understanding, and that's only a few steps away from resolving to do better.

Now, years later, I like to think that that is what I'm trying to do. Resolving to do better than when I didn't have it in me to do anything but put one foot in front of the other. Resolving to see the light in the darkness and the joy amidst the chaos. Even the kind of chaos we are currently experiencing.

So, no, I am not religious in the strict sense.

But I consider joy to be a sacred thing.

I hold it close to my chest whenever it's within reach. I look for it whenever it's missing. *Better days are coming*, I whisper with the hushed devotion these church steps call for. *Hope is a religious thing*, I sing.

Hoping against all odds is an act of devotion.

Light shining in through the cracks is a holy act of grace.

I hold both so dearly, and in my own way, pray to them often. I'll look for them today and tomorrow and until we can feel safe again. I'll look for them in everything I see.

III.

Someone recently asked me to name the biggest change I'd undergone in the past year. I saw fireworks behind my eyelids, and the kind of pain that I somehow thought I could avoid in a lifetime living fresh beneath my bones. Still cutting, still pulsing. An intermittent, constant reminder.

But I saw something else, too.

The mess at my feet, and the willingness to stay. To clean it up.

The itch to take flight, and the strength to stay put for once in my goddamn life.

The mirage of a promised high or maybe even the reality of it, and the choice to fight like hell for it.

The knowledge that the woman I was a year ago wouldn't have known how to do it. So I owe it to her to try. Because for the first time in my life, I might get to witness an impossible thing: how to accept whatever lives on and only break off little bits of it without having to throw the whole thing away.

Some nights, when I can't sleep and my feet feel heavy, I whisper to myself what I've probably known this whole time: I believe in the goodness of my own heart and in the bitterness of these lonely months; I believe in hardship, and resilience, and people. I believe things will get easier, or perhaps we'll go easier on ourselves, or perhaps the world will. I've learned to trust gut instinct over all else. I count to five, my hand on my chest. I tell myself, not yet not yet not yet not yet not yet.

But we're getting there.

On those nights, my own voice sounds like what I imagine a heart cracked open would feel like or, alternatively, the crackle before a kiss, the last dance before the music stops, raindrops on a moving glass surface, pitch black-purple sparks with a yellow centre, this goddamn city and every goddamn poetic feeling I've ever had about it.

IV.

Gloria Steinem once said, 'Marx and Engels were really nice guys, but they made one big mistake: the end doesn't justify the means. The means *are* the ends. The means create the ends that we're going to get. So if we want humour, love, good food and dancing at the end – then we want humour, love, good food and dancing along the way. Otherwise we will never get it. And we'll burn out on the way.'

Which is to say, it's up to us to not lose sight of the fire.

Whatever that means for you – ripe tomatoes, bad poetry, a flock of pigeons coming for your chocolate bar. Singing in the shower, sleeping all weekend, calling friends you haven't heard from in a while. Working hard and respecting boundaries and trying your best. Fresh fruit and cold lemonade and the beat of our own hearts. One foot in front of the other.

Just don't lose the fire.

Because we would have given up a long time ago if it weren't for all the good stuff that lives in between. And we're almost there. Or we might be, which is good enough. If we're lucky, we'll get all the time in the world once we get there. There will be hardship, and there will be humour, love, good food and dancing along the way. You're all invited. I can't wait.

– A Lot of Puking & A Lot of Magic –

The beginning

It's mid-November 2020, and the outside world is looking bleak. The pandemic is raging, it's now cold and flu season, and many people in the US have continued to argue and defy science in place of doing what needs to be done to protect one another. Covid numbers are soaring, and the upcoming holidays are set to make it all worse. My husband, Dash, and I are in southern Utah, car camping. We have just finished the first of a five-day road trip across the country to hunker down for some time with my parents in Ohio. We don't honestly know if travelling now is the right thing to be doing, but we are committed and well on our way. Hotels do not feel safe, and restaurants don't either, so we've opted to pack all our meals and sleep on a mattress in the back of our car. We will interact with as few people as possible as we travel the next 2,000 plus miles from CA. Life is ... weird.

When the sun goes down that first night in the woods, it is a lot colder than we expected and planned for, so at 6.00 pm we're already in bed. We are huddled together for warmth under layers of covers and looking up at a clear night sky through the window in the back of our Prius. It is quiet, romantic and beautiful here. I feel calm wash over me. Out there the rest of the world is in chaos, but here I feel safe. There's truly nowhere else I'd rather be on this night. It's been a great day and, aside from the chill, we are both surprisingly comfortable in our car cocoon. Our bodies are tired from hiking the nearby pink sand dunes at sunset. Our dog is lying between us to keep herself warm.

All day, we've been driving, singing, talking, re-connecting. Occasionally pausing our podcasts to daydream together, and most often today about our future children. About how fun it will be to take them on road trips, and about how ready we feel to start this next chapter. At one point this afternoon, I looked in the rear-view mirror and imagined them sitting there. My babies. I swear I could hear sibling-like laughter from the backseat.

Lying in our car bed that night, eyes already heavy at 6.00 pm, I have an overwhelming feeling that we are not far from meeting our first.

I lock eyes with my husband.

'I really want to get pregnant. With every fibre of my being, I want to have a baby next year.'

I look back up at the sky.

'I do, too,' he says. 'I'm ready. We're ready.'

And then, like magic, the most enormous shooting star dances directly above us across the night sky. It reminds me of the 'The More You Know' commercial from when I was young, that big rainbow star soaring across the TV. It glides from one end of the horizon all the way to the other. Slowly, with ease, taking its time. If I hadn't seen it, I would not believe it.

There they are, we decide, saying hello. As if to say, 'I'm ready too, Mom! I'm on my way, Dad!' Yes. Flying by, there's our baby, our babies. We thank the tiny spirits for gifting us such a beautiful sign, and then, with the – equally magic – help of our sleeping pills, float off to sleep.

New Year

Opening the garbage, I pull out the day-old, used pee stick still wrapped up in toilet paper. I've run in to look at the brand so that I might go buy another of the same kind. I've had past mishaps with other versions, and this one seems to me now the most foolproof. I pull it out and unwrap it, but today it looks different. Two lines have appeared where only one was last night. 'Ah, yes, patience,' I think. My first lesson in parenting.

I quickly run to my husband; now he sees them

too. Those two subtle lines that weren't both there last night. Those two soft pink lines that would dictate our year. Two little lines, changing our lives forever.

I am pregnant.

The date is 1 January 2021. It's New Year's Day, which, as it turns out – pandemic or not – is a pretty perfect day to find out that you will be parents. On this first day of the year, a sense of hope fills the air. As if anything is possible.

Because it is.

And it was.

Winter

There is a selfie on my phone dated 16 January. I am holding a bubbly water, pack of crackers and, having just thrown up, am smiling widely at the camera, holding up my thumb.

I am so happy to be sitting there on that early morning, hanging over a toilet bowl.

This won't be bad, I naively, foolishly, think to myself.

I have no idea what is coming.

I have no idea that the next four plus months of my life will be spent over toilet bowls.

Through spring

My doctor is kind and direct, and just who I've

needed this year. When I meet her, I am already crying. I have just stepped on a scale to learn that I am very quickly moving in the wrong direction as far as my pregnancy weight goes. While I have been told over and over again recently that morning sickness is 'common, a good sign, and very normal', I *am* also positive that losing 10lbs in two weeks is not the most healthy way to kick off a pregnancy.

I feel awful.

I look awful.

A new prescription from an Emergency Room visit last week is the only thing keeping the water I've stomached earlier from coming back up.

Dash had to leave class to drive me to my appointment this morning. This week he has also picked me up off the bathroom floor, helped me shower and put on my shoes. The nausea is constant. Whatever this is, this extreme sport of 'very normal' morning sickness, I know that I can't sustain it.

'I cannot keep doing this,' I say to my doctor.

'No you cannot,' she replies, and hands me a tissue. 'I promise that I'm going to help. We will figure this out.'

And because angels are real, and our healthcare workers are heroes, over the next few weeks of appointments, she does.

HG and me

Hyperemesis gravidarum (HG) is defined as severe nausea and vomiting during pregnancy. Through research, finding support online and seeking out other women's stories to feel less alone, it becomes clear that what I've been experiencing is considered a more mild, or moderate, case. I haven't been hospitalised overnight and I don't need a feeding tube. I have lost only 10lbs, while some women lose 60lbs. I am not at risk of losing my life, as other women most certainly are with HG. No, I will definitely survive this and I'm getting through it.

I am just, in a word, miserable.

Up to this point, my year has involved throwing up every day. On the good days it is five or six times, on the worst of the days I lose count at fifteen. I've spent all year in my bed. On the more stressful mornings, when I need to leave home, a combination of two different medications is the only way I get through. And one of them makes me grumpy and anxious.

I shake from exhaustion, feel dizzy, have a constant migraine, and because often I do not feel physically able to make it to the bathroom, there are ready-to-go-in-an-instant puke bags hanging on our bed frame. My husband has also taped down all of the curtains to block out any light. I lie down in my shower, puke in the car and worry that the baby is getting what they need, day … after day … after day.

Reading is impossible and screens all emit light, so at first I mostly just lie in the darkness. At some point I decide to have something play in the background, as to not go too crazy with only my thoughts.

I have already listened to the entire series of *Friends* and have moved on now to *Modern Family*. Occasionally, turning my head to watch a scene I remember and love.

This helps pass the time.

Once every few days I attempt a walk, to exercise, hearing over and over again just how important it is for the health of the baby. However, every yoga class (on Zoom, as we are still very much in a raging pandemic) is cut short by needing to run out of the room to get sick. And I have already left trails of vomit in most of our neighbours' front yards. Dash and I do get a good laugh at just how many of them have seen me throw up on their Ring apps.

Weeks turn into months, and I lie there and daydream about being past twenty weeks. I pray that I am in the half of women with HG whose symptoms and sickness trail off around then. And knowing that time does pass is really the only thing that I have to hold on to.

I lie on my side, rub my stomach and whisper, 'I love you, baby. I love you, baby.'

The end of the beginning

It's August. I am thirty-six weeks pregnant and sitting in the same lobby where I've sat over and over again throughout all of this year. I glance around at the other women in the room. Masked up, without partners, some likely trying not to get sick. Most look to be at the start of their pregnancy journeys. They will get good news, and scary news, have their blood drawn 300 times, and pee in those tiny cups at every damn visit here.

I have had really unpleasant times in this waiting area, but today feels very different.

Peaceful. Calm. Comforting.

Like the final satisfying chapter in a wild and unpredictable book.

I feel good. I feel strong. I am thrilled and ready to soon meet my baby.

Sitting here now, I cannot honestly remember the last time I threw up. At some point in the last few weeks of my pregnancy, the letters HG were replaced with GD, and the thoughts and worries of my day took another direction. Gestational

Diabetes (GD) is no picnic, but it has been nothing compared to HG.

I scan the room again and catch one of the women staring right back at me. I am clearly the most pregnant person in this room. I used to stare at that woman too, longing, wondering, what must that be like? To know you're so close to life changing forever. I smile at her, not yet visibly pregnant, and wonder if she currently feels sick and nauseous.

I think about January, February, March, April. Seasons changing and my feeling better and better. I remember those darker days but, also, I feel myself already forgetting.

I've just had an ultrasound and am waiting now to see the doctor. The baby looks great. There are zero concerns. All is as it should be. I remember my early weeks mantra, touch my belly, and think, 'I love you, baby. I love you, baby.' Happy tears fill my eyes. My name is called, and I quickly wipe them away.

I am proud of myself.

I am proud of my body.

I am already enamoured, and so proud of this baby.

GEORDIE STEWART

– A Journey Around My Bedroom –

February 2020 | A response to the 1794 book,
Voyage Autour de ma Chambre,
by Xavier de Maistre

I hold down the handle before gently easing the latch into its home for the night. It's late. It's usually late when I finally close the door; the norm for someone whose mind awakens when the sun sleeps. It is, however, abnormal for the rest of the household. I hope others don't hear the handle returning to its horizontal position. The only light is the deep yellow glow from the bedside lamp. At this time, it's uplighting, not down; it's time for cerebral calm not chaos.

My clothing rack fits snugly against the wall, as though it was engineered for the space available. The clothes themselves are reassuring memories: presents, parties, parades. Hanging alongside each other are formal and informal, work and pleasure, as though the clothes themselves are caught between making a life and living it.

The wooden chest stoically remains at the foot of my bed. A still-unnamed weather-beaten teddy bear sits awkwardly amongst the white pillowcases; the buoyancy of his youth replaced by fuzzy fur and a solitary eye. His adolescent yearning is camouflaged by a dull beige shade and grey wisps.

My chest of drawers, so overwhelming looking up when I was child, now requires a gentle hamstring stretch and bowed head to access the bulging lower drawer. Once again, I pull off a wooden knob. 'I must get that fixed,' I think to myself. I've been saying the same thing for years. Having returned from my cycle, I gave it a yank and the same knob rolled around the floor hopelessly. The familiarity provided a smile and confirmed it won't be fixed anytime soon.

Assorted items are dotted around the window sill and shelves: mugs, knives, medals, pens, lighters, carvings, coasters. Each has a place; each has a reason. Each fears it will join former items that have met their fate in the attic, charity shop or rubbish bin. For now, to their relief, their presence serves an unidentified purpose.

Chris's painting drags my mind to a different phase of life; one of passion and focus. *The* Chris? I smirk. So much has changed and yet also so little. It sits above the 'Geordie' room sign: inescapably innocent, irrefutably significant. The faded red carpet takes me to Morocco with Harry, the

Nicaraguan water horn to junior officer antics, Dorje's silk scarf to Everest Base Camp.

Finally, the bookshelf. Perhaps a true representation of my bedroom: a time capsule to whenever and wherever my memories want to go. A rough, random and insightful window into my past, present and future.

Close the handle and meaningful parts of my life are all there. This is my bedroom of now but largely of a life gone by and another to follow. From childhood to adulthood and boy to man, the room itself is a journey to a destination I cannot foresee.

– *Extract from* Berlin:
The Story of a City –

Experiences of bombing raids in the Second World War

Inevitably Berliners started to live part of their lives underground. Night-time activity had virtually stopped anyway, the black-out making movement dangerous and every street being patrolled by the officious police and security services. Life in the air-raid shelters began to assume its own pattern, communities forming in the cellars and stations where people spent most nights:

> 'Shuffling feet. Suitcases banging into things. Lutz Lehmann screaming "Mutti!" [Mummy]. To get to the basement shelter we have to cross the street to the side-entrance, climb down some stairs, then go along a corridor and across a square courtyard with stars overhead and aircraft buzzing like hornets. Then down some more stairs, through more doors and corridors. Finally, we're in our shelter, behind an iron door that weighs a hundred pounds. The official term is air-raid shelter. We call it cave, underworld, catacomb of fear, mass grave.'

The shelters were initially well organised but became, in themselves, something of a demonstration of how the regime began to fail as the war progressed. Many were extensions to the U-Bahn stations. They were all meant to have 2 metres of concrete and be steel-lined, but most only had a single metre despite Goebbels's assurances. The allocation was meant to be one person per square metre but again, as the bombing increased and the pressure of numbers grew, most became badly overcrowded. No provision was made for the hundreds of thousands of slave labourers imported into the city to work on the defence systems and in the factories; they were expendable. It is estimated that 12,000 German companies used slave labour in some form, many of the slave workers being Russian prisoners who after the war were told by the Soviets they should never have allowed themselves to be taken and were marched off to the Gulags. Ventilation systems were introduced so that capacity could be increased but they too were often inadequate.

In January 1946 schoolgirls in Prenzlauer Berg were asked to write an essay about their experiences in an air-raid shelter. 'The room is full of chatter and laughter,' wrote one:

'But over everything lies a nerve-shattering tension. There, a close hit! The anti-aircraft guns begin to fire. The shocks become stronger and stronger. The chatter grows softer, and the laughter stops altogether. Suddenly, a deafening bang! The lights flicker, the room sways. Frightened, we all flinch. The old woman across from me begins praying softly. Sobbing, a child buries its head in its mother's lap. Its whining hangs in the air like the embodiment of our fear. Hit after hit! Each of us feels the nearness of death. Perhaps in three minutes, perhaps two, perhaps only one! The young woman next to me stares with dull eyes into the emptiness. Like all of us, she has given up on life.'

ROBERT WILLIS

– No Room at the Inn –
A Christmas Carol

Hard was the journey and crowded the pathways
As Joseph for Mary sought shelter that night,
For Galilee's home fires seemed far, far behind them
When Bethlehem's lamps through the hills came
in sight.
Wearily, wearily, onward to Bethlehem
Seeking a welcome and comfort within;
But voices there met them with no word
of greeting
And stark was the message: 'No room at the Inn.'

Over earth's pathways the people are moving
By will of great Caesar compelled to leave home,
From valley and village in Syrian landscapes
The people are moving, commanded to roam.
Wearily, wearily, onward to Bethlehem
Hoping as night falls some shelter to win,
But lamplight and firelight give false hope
of welcome
The doors close against them: 'No room at
the Inn.'

Through the bleak darkness comes one sound
    of welcome,
A voice giving promise of shelter and rest,
Some kindly words spoken, a stable door opened,
To find there a manger as birds find their nest.
Cheerily, cheerily, home now in Bethlehem
Where for the Christ child new life must begin,
For one voice of welcome, enough for
    God's purpose,
Is saying no longer: 'No room at the Inn.'

– *Extract from* The Art of Exploration: Lessons in Curiosity, Leadership and Getting Things Done –

The importance of self-awareness

The year 2020 will be remembered as the Great Pause. As the world went into lockdown, billions of people were quarantined in their own homes for weeks and months on end due to the coronavirus pandemic. For thousands across the globe it was a time of tragedy, losing loved ones to this terrible disease. For many millions more it was financially ruinous, as jobs and businesses went under and the economy plummeted.

Of course, it affected many people in different ways, but despite its awful impact and terrible consequences, if we were to fathom some positives to come out of the whole mess, it would be fair to say that it brought many communities together, unified in purpose and a desire to help one another get through it. Perhaps even more importantly, it forced a great number of us to take stock and reflect on our lives in a way that we never have before. It certainly did for me.

It is quite remarkable what a few weeks of solitary confinement can do for you. Shakespeare wrote *King Lear* while quarantining from the plague and the playhouses were closed, and the famous seventeenth-century diarist Samuel Pepys documented the impact of the rampant 1665 bubonic plague in London:

> But, Lord! how sad a sight it is to see the streets empty of people, and very few upon the 'Change. Jealous of every door that one sees shut up, lest it should be the plague; and about us two shops in three, if not more, generally shut up.

Seclusion has also afforded a great many writers over the centuries the chance to come up with their finest masterpieces. Dante wrote *The Divine Comedy* whilst in exile, and Cervantes came up with *Don Quixote* whilst behind bars. Dostoyevsky too was inspired to write two of his finest works after spending months in jail, and let's not forget Nelson Mandela, and a whole host of other political leaders. It seems that having one's liberty removed temporarily, if looked at with a positive mindset, can enable you to focus on things that really matter; and that begins with self-reflection and an understanding of oneself.

I am certain that, in time, we will look back at 2020 as being a year of catalytic change in many ways – politically, economically, and socially. We have lived through historic times, and I believe that much of the change to come will be driven by people who have used the time wisely, thinking about what they can do to improve themselves. There are the obvious things that many of us aspire to, such as reading books, getting fit, learning an instrument or a new language, or perhaps taking up a new hobby, whether that's origami or baking. But as well as the 'easy wins', I'm also referring to deep, fundamental changes in how we go about our daily lives, committing ourselves to a new regime of betterment in how we treat ourselves and others – and all this begins with understanding.

I've heard more than one person say that – if not for the losses that so many people have suffered – they were almost glad the pandemic happened, because it gave them the first chance of a break in their lives for decades. If it takes a coronavirus to give you the time to do what you want in life, then that would suggest a strong case for examining how you live; and you can only do that if you are self-aware. We can make big changes at any point in our lives, but we often get distracted because of work, relationships and other external factors, and it is easy to ignore what is happening deep inside of us. As well as taking care of our physical health, we need to carve out time to work on our self-awareness.

There are few times in our lives when we are forced to be still and make peace with our decisions, because we have no choice but to do otherwise. For me as an explorer and professional traveller, the year 2020 was the first time in over a decade that I'd spent more than a couple of months in one place, so it was certainly a big change from the norm.

At first I remember feeling trapped and a bit claustrophobic, stuck in London when all I wanted was to enjoy the freedom of the road. All my trips got cancelled and, like many freelancers, I lost an entire year's worth of wages. It was made harder by the fact that I ended up breaking an ankle, which forced me to stay put, even if there was a temptation at times to escape. It would have been simple to just sit in front of the TV and do nothing, but, instead of moping, I decided to try and use the time wisely and write down some of the lessons I have learned from travel, and in doing so reflect on what I could do better.

It reminded me of the last time I was forced to stay still and take stock in the summer of 2015. It was under slightly different circumstances, but with a rather similar outcome. I remember the date well – it was 19 August. I was on an expedition in the Himalayas, when the taxi I was travelling in took a tumble off the edge of a cliff in the dead of night, and I was plunged into a jungle ravine. Somehow I survived and escaped that time with only a broken arm and a few smashed ribs, but I ended up having to halt the journey for fifty days while I recovered from the accident. I'm sure a close brush with death is enough to give anyone pause for thought, and it forced me to re-evaluate things and ask myself a few questions about my own life, who I was, and where I was going.

Quite often we can get on a path to reach a 'destination', but neglect to re-evaluate the next stage once we get there: we simply keep going in the same direction without thinking. This can happen in business, relationships or in any part of our life. How often do you sit back and think – *really think* – about whether or not the path you are on is the right one? Maybe it was the right choice for you a few years ago, but life changes us, and what works for the person you were *then*, may not be right for the person you are *now*.

SUSIE CORETH

– Be Still, My Restless Mind –

If stillness be the mind at peace
    And restlessness can ever cease,
If calmness be the utmost goal
And streams of thought that tire the soul
Can end, I am in want; I seek
A way to still a mind that's weak
To spins: it is a thought cyclone,
It hunts for roughened paths to roam,
It turns and twists, it's high, it's low,
It's reckless in its restless show,
Erratic, up and side to side,
Constantly swimming against the tide;
It's fitful, jumping all over the place,
From happy to sad, from earth to space,
It wants to run away, be wild;
It is a drifting, fidgety child
Longing to find a place to play
To while away a disruptive day,
The child wants windswept fields, trees
And sky-blue reflections on rippling seas,
Wants mountain paths on which to climb;
That child holds on to this restless mind.

Wandering, lost or not lost at all
But searching, seeking a purpose, a call,
Or not seeking, but hoping for something else –
A different path, a greater self.
Is there an answer? What do I need?
Are you, my mind, just full of greed
For all things in this beautiful world,
So remain in this restless swirl?
Be still, I ask, be quiet and still,
To contemplate my heart at will
And not get lost amongst the crowd
Of thoughts that scream so very loud.
And yet, they are my beating heart,
They are my paints, they are my art,
And in the alcoves, buried deep
This artwork's purely mine to keep,
It may be rotten, rough with dirt,
Filled with colour enriched with hurt,
But this canvas (once loved by me),
Shall hold my self eternally,
Up and down in painted thought,
Perpetual onslaught, stop; I ought
To throw this canvas that I find
And still my restless mind.
Only in stillness will I find
A way to calm my restless mind,
The mind in need of compassion and peace

And yet the butterflies won't cease,
Or will they? A moment of quiet. And then
The vultures are ready to fly again,
An endless cycle, a dreamer's curse,
Though, in truth, there's so much worse;
How lucky to have a mind that's free
To go wherever it wants to be,
Quite so, how fortunate am I,
My mind dances 'cross starlit skies,
I'll let it dance all through the night,
Come morning, it'll be alright.
Come morning, it'll be alright,
It dances more in darkened night,
Dancing, sleepless, thoughts, time,
Be still, my ever-restless mind,
Perpetuate a kinder self,
Put doubts forever on the shelf
And any negativity:
You are of no use to me.
Calmness, I will find, be kind,
Be still, my restless mind.

– Authors' Biographies –

Olivia Acland – Olivia Acland is the *Economist*'s correspondent in central Africa, based in eastern Democratic Republic of the Congo (DRC). She has spent five years in Africa and writes on a range of topics from cheesemaking to rap music, politics, mining and insect farming. She has covered elections in DRC, Congo Brazzaville, Sierra Leone and Burundi. She also takes photos for Reuters. She has a dog called Stella and a goat called Nelson.

Charly Afia – Charly Afia is an actress who grew up in Ghana and Surrey. She has a passion for nature, wildlife and being outdoors.

Sarah Agha – Sarah Agha read Theology at Trinity College Dublin before returning to London to pursue acting. She has performed with the Royal Shakespeare Company and her TV credits include *Homeland*, *Into The Badlands* and *SAS: Rogue Heroes*. She also works regularly as a voiceover artist and writes for *Backstage* magazine.

Jenna Al-Ansari – Jenna Al-Ansari is a Bahraini/British writer, living in London. She won the inaugural Screenshot competition in 2021 and is developing her winning entry, *Protect & Survive*, with Sister Pictures and South Of The River. Jenna's original television series, *The Moderators*, is currently in development with Hat Trick Productions. Jenna also works with OKRE and The Wellcome Trust, supporting the development of television, video games and films which contribute to a better understanding of subjects such as planetary emergency, mental health, poverty and migration.

Chloë Ashby – Chloë Ashby is an author and arts journalist. Since graduating from the Courtauld Institute of Art, she has written for the *TLS*, the *Guardian*, the *FT Life & Arts*, *frieze*, amongst others. Her first non-fiction book, *Look At This If You Love Great Art*, was published in June 2021. Her debut novel, *Wet Paint*, is due in April 2022.

Derren Brown – Derren Brown has re-defined magic through his TV and stage events, exhilarating audiences worldwide with a unique brand of mind-control, suggestion, showmanship and illusion. Through his award-winning shows he has gained a reputation as a performer prepared to constantly challenge and break down boundaries. He is also a best-selling author and accomplished painter.

Harry Bucknall – Harry Bucknall, who once served in the British Army, delights in classical travel and especially long journeys, be they by ferry through the Greek Islands, walking the pilgrimage from London to Rome or travelling around Britain, the subject of his latest book, *A Road for All Seasons*, due for publication in summer 2022.

Melkon Charchoglyan – Melkon Charchoglyan is a writer, translator and photographer from Armenia, living in London. He is the 2021 Helen Deutsch Fellow at Boston University, Massachusetts, where he writes and teaches fiction.

Alice Church – Alice Church is a writer and historian based in Dorset. Since graduating from University College London in 2012, she has worked on various historical writing projects and had her first book, a biography of Lady Georgiana Lennox, published in 2016. Her second book, a historical fiction titled *The Belles of Waterloo*, will be published in 2022. This anthology includes Alice's first published short story, inspired by her move to the countryside during the 2020 lockdown.

Mark Coreth – Mark Coreth is a sculptor of the natural world, adventurer, private pilot and former soldier. Mark travels to the harshest parts of the world to study and understand the wildlife that he creates in bronze, his aeroplane often being his chariot!

Susie Coreth – Susie Coreth was brought up in the countryside in Wiltshire before studying at the University of St Andrews and the International School of Screen Acting. She is a writer, actress and filmmaker. She performed her play, *Ivory Wings*, at the Edinburgh Fringe and in London to sell-out audiences. She is currently writing her first novel and running a film recommendation account @a_different_film, which she started at the beginning of the pandemic to inspire people to discover something new and unexpected.

Frances Dimond – Frances Dimond was educated at The Grey Coat Hospital and Bedford College, University of London. She had a thirty-six-year career at The Royal Archives, and the Royal Photograph Collection (as Curator) at Windsor Castle. She is currently retired and working on a biography of Queen Alexandra.

Carol Ann Duffy – Carol Ann Duffy was born in Glasgow. She grew up in Stafford and then attended the University of Liverpool, where she studied Philosophy. She has written for both children and adults, and her poetry has received many awards, including the Signal Prize for Children's Verse, the Whitbread and Forward Prizes, as well as the Lannan Literary Award and the E.M. Forster Prize in America. In 2012 she was awarded the PEN Pinter Prize. She was Poet Laureate from 2009 to 2019.

Amaryllis Earle – Amaryllis Earle is a poet based in London who discovered her writing during a difficult time battling with chronic pain throughout her twenties. She also runs her own company in the beauty technology industry, advocates for hidden disabilities and raises awareness for those living with chronic illnesses. She lives in southwest London with her husband and their rescue dog Basil.

Sophie Elwes – Sophie Elwes hosts the podcast *A Life Less Ordinary with Sophie Elwes*. When she's not working at Back Up, a spinal injuries charity, Sophie enjoys spending her time water-skiing and wakeboarding, and competes internationally.

Julian Fellowes – Julian Fellowes won the Oscar for the Best Original Screenplay in 2002 for *Gosford Park*. Since then, he has written many films, stage musicals, novels and television series, including *Downton Abbey*. The second *Downton Abbey* film was released in March 2022, and Julian is now working on *The Gilded Age* for HBO.

Tom Felton – In January 2022, Tom Felton starred in the SKY Original film *Save the Cinema*, starring opposite Samantha Morton. He collaborated twice with the BAFTA-winning director Amma Asante in the critically acclaimed period dramas *Belle* and *A United Kingdom*, starred in *Rise of the Planet of the Apes* and as Draco Malfoy in the *Harry Potter* films.

Richard Frazer – Richard Frazer is minister of Greyfriars Kirk, Edinburgh. He founded the Grassmarket Community Project, supporting people on the edge of society, and the Greyfriars Charteris Centre, promoting wellbeing, inclusive community and social enterprise. He has written about and been involved in reviving pilgrimage in Scotland after centuries of Protestant opposition.

Stephanie Greenwood – Born in London, Stephanie Greenwood grew up in South Africa and France, before studying at Dartmouth College (USA). Among other acting credits, she has written two plays: *It's Beautiful Over There* (Edinburgh Fringe

Festival, Tristan Bates Theatre) and *Relative Motion*. She is co-director of theatre company Very Rascals and is currently completing her MA (Acting) at the Royal Conservatoire of Scotland.

Joshua Levine – Joshua Levine is an author and historian. He has written extensively about twentieth-century history. He lives in London with his wife, daughter and cat.

Alexander McCall Smith – Alexander McCall Smith's books have been translated into over forty-six languages and have sold more than 30 million copies across the world. These include *The No. 1 Ladies' Detective Agency* series, the *44 Scotland Street* novels and the *Isabel Dalhousie* series, as well as stand-alone novels, poetry and children's fiction.

Leon McCarron – Leon McCarron's words come from slow, immersive journeys. He has travelled over 35,000 miles on foot and by bike and boat, and tells stories big and small through the voices of those on the ground. His third book, *Wounded Tigris: A River Journey Through the Cradle of Civilisation*, will be published in late 2022.

Anna Myers – Anna Myers is a writer, voiceover artist and creative consultant. She's written about identity, culture, lifestyle and everything in between for publications such as *Teen Vogue*, *Elle*, *Refinery29*, *Glamour*, *Grazia* and many more. She writes a newsletter about the joys of building a life and is on Instagram @annamyers139

Katherine Skelton – Katherine Skelton is an actor and writer based in Los Angeles. Favourite TV and film acting credits include *Angie Tribeca*, *Community*, *Scandal*, *House of Lies* and *Super Troopers 2*. Most recently, Katherine co-wrote, produced, acted in and directed the short form digital series *Grow The F*ck Up*, which you can watch at gtfuseries.com

Geordie Stewart – Geordie Stewart is an author, explorer, mountaineer and former British Army officer. He was the youngest Briton to climb the Seven Summits – the highest mountain on each of the seven continents – and has completed a 22,500-mile solo cycle around the world.

Barney White-Spunner – Barney White-Spunner is a historian and former soldier. His book, *Berlin: The Story of a City*, published widely across four continents, was born from a deep fascination and love for this extraordinary city.

Robert Willis – Robert Willis has been Dean of Canterbury since 2001. He had served as Dean of Hereford since 1992. Music has been a lifelong hobby and his hymns and words for songs and carols have been a constant interest. Canterbury Cathedral is a place of pilgrimage, the Mother Church of Anglicans worldwide and a World Heritage Site. It is also a constant gathering place for groups from all nations.

Levison Wood – Levison Wood is an award-winning author, explorer and photographer who specialises in documenting people and cultures in remote regions and post-conflict zones. He has published nine best-selling books and produced a number of critically acclaimed documentaries, which have been aired around the world.

Information about Shout 85258

Shout 85258 is a free, confidential, 24/7 text messaging support service for anyone in the UK who is struggling to cope. Text 'SHOUT' to 85258 at any time of the day or night to speak to a trained volunteer.

Shout 85258 supports children, young people and adults across the UK experiencing any type of mental health concern, including anxiety, stress, depression, suicidal thoughts and self-harm. People also text us for support with isolation and loneliness, grief, bullying, relationship challenges, sexual identity, eating and body issues, substance misuse and abuse.

As a digital service, Shout was one of the only mental health support services able to operate as normal during the Covid-19 pandemic and more people than ever turned to us. We take around 1,400 conversations every day with people in need of immediate support with their mental health.

Shout is powered by charity Mental Health Innovations and was developed with the support of the Royal Foundation as a legacy of its Heads Together campaign.

Shout is there around the clock for those needing 'in the moment' support. Just £10 pays for a conversation that could save a life.

– Acknowledgements –

There are so many people who helped create *Out of Isolation*, for whom I'm incredibly grateful. First and foremost, thank you to all the authors for writing such fascinating pieces and donating them to this anthology. It is nothing without you.

To the team at Unicorn Publishing Group, in particular Lord Strathcarron, who took a chance on this book when it was just an idea, and to Ramona Lamport, Felicity Price-Smith, Lauren Tanner and Vivian Head for your brilliant work bringing it to life. Thank you also to Alice Church for your words of advice and for putting me in contact with Ian.

Thank you to Felicity Brown and Lisa Gilbert at Mental Health Innovations for your guidance and assistance in enabling this anthology to raise money for Shout 85258.

My heartfelt thanks to Jamie Lonsdale, Sarah Elwes and Sophie Elwes for your generous financial support and kindness. To all those who donated to the crowdfund campaign, a special thank you. In particular, Sophie Fernandes, Natalie Norman and David Cox.

Finally, an enormous thank you to my parents, Seonaid and Mark Coreth, my siblings Jamie, Anna and Freddie, and also to Will Frazer and Francesca FitzHerbert for completing our lockdown family. You all kept me going during the pandemic and this anthology wouldn't be here without your support, advice, ideas, creativity and laughter.

Susie Coreth, February 2022